MW00389293

A Guide to
Technical Consulting
for the Clinical
Laboratory

CATHY L. MANSKE

Strategic Book Publishing and Rights Co.

Strategic Book Publishing and Rights Co.
12620 FM 1960, Suite A4-507
Houston, TX 77065
www.sbpra.com

ISBN: 978-1-62212-699-6

Interior Book Design: Judy Maenle

Dedication

I dedicate this guide to the medical technologists who spent four years earning a Bachelor of Science degree in medical technology only to discover that a CLA (certified laboratory assistant) or MLT (medical laboratory technician) with only two years (or less) of education could be hired to do your job. I hope after reading this guide you will find it beneficial and be encouraged and motivated to use your education and experience to pursue a fulfilling and rewarding profession as a clinical laboratory technical consultant.

The biggest benefit to becoming a technical consultant is that *you* are in charge! *You* can choose your own hours, *you* can determine your own work schedule, and *you* can decide when to take time off because *you are not* tethered to a workplace! If you choose to work as an independent technical consultant, *you* can also determine your income, say good-bye to working holidays and weekends, double shifts, and crazy shifts, and you'll no longer have to deal with hospital politics. Sound enticing? Read on, and welcome aboard!

Acknowledgments

It is with deep love and gratitude that I acknowledge the ongoing support, advice, and editing expertise from my husband, Neal, without whose encouragement this airplane would never have left the ground.

I also would like to acknowledge the following people whose professional knowledge and help made it possible for me to write this guide:

Denise Barbeau, Program Manager
Arizona Department of Health Services
Division of Public Health Services
Bureau of Laboratory Services

Marcie Bentley, CLIA Surveyor
Arizona Department of Health Services
Division of Public Health Services
Bureau of Laboratory Services

Kathy Nucifora, Accreditation Manager
COLA

Sandra Laughlin, MT (ASCP), Product Manager
CompuGroup Medical US

Table of Contents

Preface

The purpose in writing this guide is to offer consulting guidance, based on my personal experiences, and to provide regulatory instruction to qualified individuals, especially medical technologists, who want to pursue a career as a technical consultant. However, because laboratory science programs do not, to my knowledge, offer classes in the interpretation and application of clinical laboratory regulations or technical consulting, interested candidates do not have the education or training to become professionals in the special field of technical consulting for a clinical laboratory or for a physician's office laboratory (POL).

This guide also has a selfish purpose. I hope it will help others to forge into technical consulting and allow me to eventually transition into retirement! Then, hopefully, I can extract myself from the laboratories I serve, and hand the baton over to a new and qualified person who has read, and is ready to apply, the information presented in this guide.

DISCLAIMER: The regulatory compliance, applications, and enforcements of the Clinical Laboratory Improvement Amendments of 1988 (CLIA) regulations mentioned in this guide are based on my experiences working with Arizona's Department of Health Services, Division of Public Health Services, and the Office of Laboratory Services. Therefore, it is important for readers to understand that they might experience individual state regulatory compliance, applications, and enforcements of CLIA regulations differently.

Even though the CLIA rules and regulations governing clinical laboratories are federal government rules and regulations, their application and enforcement can be altered by each state, so long as they meet or exceed the federal requirements. For example, California requires that all clinical laboratory-testing personnel must have a California license issued by the California Department of Public Health in order to perform testing. New York and Washington states are actually CLIA exempt because they have stringent state rules of their own.

For a complete listing of state agencies and contact information, refer to the Centers for Medicare and Medicaid Services (CMS) website www.cms.gov/clia. Select "State Agency & Regional Office CLIA Contacts" for specific information about the application and enforcement of CLIA regulations in your state.

CHAPTER 1

What Is a Technical Consultant?

Every non-waived clinical laboratory must have a technical consultant professional, usually a medical technologist, who uses his or her education, training, and clinical laboratory experience to monitor all aspects of a clinical laboratory. In doing so, the goal is to ensure compliance with the Clinical Laboratory Improvement Amendments (CLIA) of 1988.

The diagram that follows will show several of the areas that typically require the technical consultant's oversight and management. I have shown this diagram many times to doctors and others who have asked, "What does a technical consultant do?" This diagram shows them the duties and tasks of a technical consultant and highlights the importance of the technical consultant's knowledge and application of CLIA regulations, which is a daunting subject for many doctors and administrators. In the early stages of considering an in-house laboratory, the staff should understand that CLIA is a series of federal government regulations associated with clinical laboratories and having a knowledgeable person become involved as their technical consultant would be beneficial and preferable.

The technical consultant's first priority is to calm the staff's CLIA fears, and help them establish a successful laboratory that will contribute to better patient care and the financial well-being of the doctors' medical practice.

It is worth mentioning that testing personnel are not involved in most of the tasks on the diagram. Their time is spent preparing

1

for testing, performing testing, and reporting test results—pre-analytical, analytical, and post-analytical tasks. This leaves little or no time for additional tasks. Also, since CLIA requires that testing personnel can qualify with a minimum of a high school diploma or General Equivalency Diploma (GED) these testers will have little, if any, working knowledge and experience pertaining to laboratory protocols and procedures to bring to the job. Even at the next level of education, MLT or CLA, workers have completed a laboratory science program, but they, too, will have limited knowledge and experience of these tasks. Therefore, the technical consultant's assistance is a must. Just as good businesses rely on tax accountants and attorneys for financial and legal help, medical practices need technical consultants to help with the regulatory compliances for their laboratories.

Some technical consultants are self-employed and work as independent contractors. They provide consulting services for medical practices in their cities or in nearby areas that want to start in-house laboratories. Once the laboratory has been established, they may choose to continue consulting for the medical practice to ensure the success of that laboratory though CLIA compliance.

Other technical consultants are employed by instrument manufacturing companies. Often they find themselves stretched thin because of the large geographical area they must cover. In the southwest, they often cover all of Arizona, New Mexico, Nevada, California, and Hawaii. Oftentimes, they are climbing on airplanes to conduct training sessions or to help run linearity or calibration verification studies for a client. Sometimes, a consultant's only contact with laboratory staff is by e-mail or by phone or as a technical support person who is available to help with an instrument problem or to answer questions. They are not independent consultants and, therefore, must answer to a higher authority.

Other technical consultants work for technical consultant companies that are consultant companies within larger medical supply and service companies. In this instance, the parent companies are in the business of providing a variety of medical services, including the placement of laboratory instruments, and providing laboratory reagents and supplies via their sales staff. These consultants benefit from having sales representatives within the organization who not only provide new startup leads to their technical consultants, but also work hand-in-hand with them to ensure CLIA compliance and ongoing business for the company.

LABORATORY TECHNICAL CONSULTING

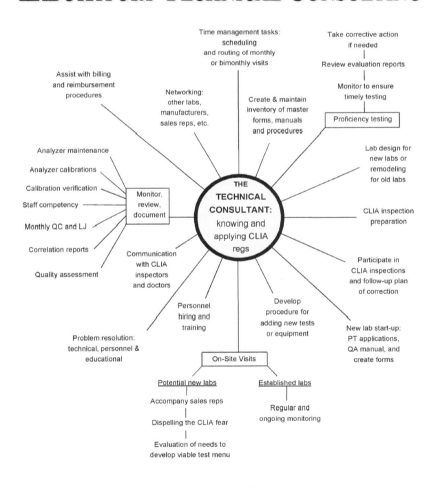

CHAPTER 2

Technical Consultant Qualifications

The federal government has developed regulations for clinical laboratories. Included in these regulations are the qualifications and job descriptions for the laboratory director, clinical consultant, testing personnel, and technical consultant.

Title 42: Public Health
Chapter IV Centers For Medicare & Medicaid Services,
Department Of Health And Human Services
Part 493: Laboratory Requirements
Subpart M: Personnel for Non-waived Testing
§493.1411 Standard; Technical consultant qualifications

The laboratory must employ one or more individuals who are qualified by education and either training or experience to provide technical consultation for each of the specialties and subspecialties of service in which the laboratory performs moderate complexity tests or procedures. The director of a laboratory performing moderate complexity testing may function as the technical consultant provided he or she meets the qualifications specified in this section.

The technical consultant must possess a current license issued by the State in which the laboratory is located, if such licensing is required.

The technical consultant must

(i) Be a doctor of medicine or doctor of osteopathy licensed to practice medicine or osteopathy in the State in which the laboratory is located; and

(ii) Be certified in anatomic or clinical pathology, or both, by the American Board of Pathology or the American Osteopathic Board of Pathology or possess qualifications that are equivalent to those required for such certification; or

(i) Be a doctor of medicine, doctor of osteopathy, or doctor of podiatric medicine licensed to practice medicine, osteopathy, or doctor of podiatry in the State in which the laboratory is located; and

(ii) Have one year of laboratory training or experience, or both in non-waived testing, in the designated specialty or subspecialty areas of service for which the technical consultant is responsible (for example, physicians certified either in hematology or hematology and medical oncology by the American board of Internal Medicine are qualified to serve as the technical consultant in hematology); or

(i) Hold an earned doctoral or master's degree in chemical, physical, biological or clinical laboratory science or medical technology from an accredited institution; and

(ii) Have at least one year of laboratory training or experience, or both in non-waived testing, the designated specialty or subspecialty areas of service for which the technical consultant is responsible; or

(ii) Have earned a bachelor's degree in a chemical, physical or biological science or medical technology from an accredited institution;

(ii) Have at least 2 years of laboratory training or experience, or both in non-waived testing, in the designated specialty or subspecialty areas of service for which the technical consultant is responsible.

Note: The technical consultant requirements for "laboratory training or experience, or both" in each specialty or subspecialty may be acquired concurrently in more than one of the specialties or subspecialties of service, excluding waived tests. For example, an individual who has a bachelor's degree in biology and additionally has documentation of two years of work experience performing tests of moderate complexity in all specialties and subspecialties of service would be qualified as a technical consultant in a laboratory performing moderate complexity testing in all specialties and subspecialties of service. [57 FR 7172, Feb. 28, 1992, as amended at 58 FR 5234, Jan. 19, 1993]

CHAPTER 3

Technical Consultant Job Description

The technical consultant is responsible for the quality aspects of laboratory operations including, but not limited to, personnel evaluation, in-service and educational training, assisting in the selection of appropriate instrumentation and in the selection of test methodology. Laboratory policies should reinforce the requirement that the technical consultant carry out and document the following responsibilities.

§493.1413 Standard; Technical Consultant Responsibilities

The technical consultant is responsible for the technical and scientific oversight of the laboratory. The technical consultant is not required to be onsite at all times testing is performed; however, he or she must be available to the laboratory on an as-needed basis to provide consultation, as specified in paragraph A. of this section.

The technical consultant must be accessible to the laboratory to provide on-site, telephone, or electronic consultation; and

The technical consultant is responsible for:

Selection of test methodology appropriate for the clinical use of the test results;

Verification of the test procedures performed and the establishment of the laboratory's test performance characteristic, including the precision and accuracy of each test and test system;

Cathy L. Manske

Enrollment and participation in a HHS-approved proficiency testing program commensurate with the services offered;

Establishing a quality control program appropriate for the testing performed and establishing the parameters for acceptable levels of analytic performance and ensuring that these levels are maintained throughout the entire testing process from the initial receipt of the specimen, through sample analysis and reporting of test results;

Resolving technical problems and ensuring that remedial actions are taken whenever test systems deviate from the laboratory's established performance specification;

Ensuring that patient test results are not reported until all corrective actions have been taken and the test system is functioning properly;

Identifying training needs and assuring that each individual performing tests receives regular in-service training and education appropriate for the type and complexity of the laboratory services performed;

Evaluating the competency of all testing personnel and assuring that the staff maintain their competency to perform test procedures and report test results promptly, accurately, and proficiently;

Direct observations of routine patient test performance, including patient preparation, if applicable, specimen handling, processing and testing;

Monitoring the recording and reporting of test results;

Review of intermediate test results or worksheets, quality control records, proficiency testing results, and preventive maintenance records;

Direct observation of performance of instrument maintenance and function checks;

Assessment of test performance through testing previously analyzed specimens, internal blind testing samples or external proficiency testing samples; and

Assessment of problem solving skills; and

Evaluation and documenting the performance of individuals responsible for moderate complexity testing at least semiannually during the first year the individual tests patient specimens. Thereafter, evaluations must be performed at least annually unless test methodology or instrumentation changes, in which case, prior to reporting patient test results; the individual's performance must be re-evaluated to include the use of the new test methodology or instrumentation.

CHAPTER 4

What is CLIA?

CLIA is the widely used acronym for the Clinical Laboratory Improvement Amendments of 1988. This body of work defines the US Federal Regulatory Standards that apply to all clinical laboratory testing performed on human specimens (except for clinical trials or basic research specimens) for the purpose of providing information for the diagnosis, prevention, or treatment of disease or impairment, and for the assessment of health. An objective of CLIA is to ensure the accuracy, reliability, and timeliness of test results.

In order for a laboratory to perform testing under CLIA, it must comply with all applicable CLIA regulations. These regulations can be found on the Centers for Medicare and Medicaid Services (CMS) website www.cms.gov/clia. Compliance with these regulations is a condition of certification for the CLIA Program, which sets standards, and issues license certificates for clinical laboratory testing. Consult the CMS website for license fees that are based on the total annual test volume of a clinical laboratory.

CMS has the primary responsibility to oversee the operation of the CLIA Program. Within CMS, the program is administered by the Center for Medicaid and State Operations, Survey and Certification Group, Division of Laboratory Services. User fees collected from more than 220,000 laboratories around the country fund the CLIA Program.

CHAPTER 5

Dispelling the CLIA Fear

There seems to be a pervasive fear among doctors to become involved with CLIA. Perhaps it is because CLIA is a comprehensive federal program. They may have heard stories about laboratories being sanctioned, heavily fined, or even shut down by CLIA inspectors.

So the question becomes, "How does the technical consultant get through the door to help dispel the CLIA fear?" One way I have found to be effective is by cultivating relationships with medical supply sales representatives who call on medical practices. Let them know you are knowledgeable about CLIA and laboratory operations and that you would be willing to talk to doctors in these practices who might be interested in setting up their own lab, but have fears about CLIA. Sales representatives already call on these practices regularly and know the staff. With their help, you can ask for a meeting with key doctors and staff or offer to attend their next provider meeting. If they don't have regular meetings, suggest meeting early in the morning, later in the day, during a lunch hour, or at a time when they aren't seeing patients.

At the meeting, hand out your business card, indicate that you'd like to help dispel possible fears about CLIA, and ask if they have questions for you. Usually someone asks something about CLIA regulations. Your confidence in answering questions and sharing your knowledge of CLIA regulations will relieve apprehensions. After the staff asks you questions, you can ask them questions. Their answers will help you to learn more about their practice. Here are some questions to ask.

- What type of practice is it?
- How many doctors and practitioners are in the practice?
- Has anyone contacted any insurance companies about reimbursement payment for in-house laboratory testing? (An important first step)
- What are the most frequent lab tests sent out to reference labs?
- How many of these tests are sent out in a day? Usually five–ten chemistry panels and/or CBCs per day is the minimum to consider testing in-house.
- Who will be doing the lab testing? Will someone need to be hired to do this, or will someone in the practice do the testing?
- Who will do the insurance billing for the lab? (Important to the success of any lab)
- Where could the lab be located? A countertop and sink may be essential.

At the beginning or the end of the meeting, offer a brief history of your laboratory experiences and places you have worked. You may even have a brief biography of yourself ready to hand out. Suggest that you have a follow-up meeting to discuss their progress in answering the questions discussed and encourage them to e-mail or call you with new questions or concerns.

Usually these meetings are effective at establishing you as a valuable and knowledgeable professional. They will begin to feel more comfortable about CLIA regulations and establishing a laboratory of their own, and including you in the process.

CHAPTER 6

Getting Started as a Technical Consultant

Once you have established a relationship with a few medical sales representatives and have had a chance to meet with some key people in a few medical practices, either with the help of a sales representative or through your own contacts, you've cleared the first hurdle to getting started as a technical consultant.

The nice thing when starting out is that you can continue to work your present job and still call on a lab or two at the end of your regular workday or on your day off. This works especially well if you are finished with your primary job early in the afternoon or if you work only part time. When the doctors in a medical practice have a serious interest in having their own laboratory, they usually begin by talking to their sales representatives who in turn will talk to you. They will want to get you involved in setting up the lab because as the laboratory consultant you ensure that the lab will be monitored for CLIA compliance. Thus, it is job security for them and for you . . . a win-win relationship. Once you have one lab under your belt, more will be on the way. Sales representatives talk to other sales representatives, doctors talk to other doctors, and word of mouth will spread that you are a qualified professional and a real asset to a medical practice. Eventually, you will become busy enough to resign from your regular job, or at least drop back to part-time status.

While sales representatives can be a great resource for you, it is important to remember that you must first serve the client . . . the medical practice. Once "on board" you will be responsible to work with the practice doctors and staff as they make decisions about instrumentation, laboratory information systems, test methodology, and testing supplies. The sales representatives are often influenced by commissions, incentives from manufacturers, and by their own management staff. In some cases, options and incentives offered to doctors by salespeople may have to be evaluated. As their technical consultant, they will expect you to investigate a wide range of factors related to acquiring an instrument irrespective of what sales incentives are offered by a manufacturer. When you've reviewed all the options—monthly payment for the instrument, operating costs, and annual instrument maintenance fees—you will have important facts to suggest an appropriate test menu and analyzer. However, remember the choice is still the doctors', even after you have done your due diligence.

CHAPTER 7

Feasibility for Starting a Lab

A practice that has several practitioners (four or more) has the best potential for a successful in-house laboratory. The more doctors and practitioners in a practice the better; a doctor who has an office with only one other doctor, physician's assistant (PA), or certified nurse practitioner (CNP) might spend more money running the lab than will be recouped from payments on insurance claims. Once you've established that a practice is large enough to support a lab and that a practice is interested in moving forward with establishing a lab, you will need to discuss a possible test menu and instrumentation.

The test menu should only include the tests most frequently ordered in the practice. All too often doctors become excited about having a lab and want to do every test known to man—a bad idea. The success of a lab will be indexed off of its test volume. Something to keep in mind is once a purchase order (PO) is signed, the practice is committed to getting the instrument and making monthly payments for the term of the lease (usually three–five years). If, during that time, test volumes decrease, then reagents and test kits become outdated, and income from health insurance claims go down, leaving the practice in the red. So, for obvious reasons, it makes good sense to have several practitioners when considering having a laboratory.

An important first task in preparing for an in-house lab is for the practice administrator to contact their account representative for their reference laboratories they presently send testing to and request a test volume breakdown of tests sent to the reference laboratory for the last twelve months. Knowing the tests ordered most often and their volumes will help you assess what tests should be on the initial test menu. It's important to remember that even after a new lab is set up, some tests will still need to be sent out to a reference lab. This is determined in part by economic viability, such as test volume and by the patient's insurance carrier. I usually figure that only 65 percent of the tests sent out to reference labs will be approved for testing in-house. This is determined by the contracts the practice has with health insurance providers. Also, some insurance carriers have agreements with reference laboratories to perform their patients' tests and won't allow the practice to do any in-house lab testing.

Once you've established the menu of tests and their volumes, it's time to start researching and evaluating each instrument the lab will need in order to do the testing. For larger instruments, compare the monthly cost of buying the instrument, leasing it, or considering a reagent rental of the instrument. Consult with the sales representative to get instrument proposals that include the price of QC materials, calibrators, consumables, and the cost per reportable, *not cost per test*.

- Cost per test is the cost of the reagent divided by the number of tests that can be performed per reagent.

  Example: reagent cost is $100 ÷ 25 tests the reagent can perform = $4.00, the cost per test.

- Cost per reportable is the cost of the reagent divided by the number of tests that can be performed per reagent, *plus* the cost of running daily QC, regular calibrations, proficiency samples, and test repeats.

  Example: reagent cost is $100 ÷ 25 tests the reagent can perform + $1.00 for QC, calibrations, proficiency samples and test repeats = $5.00, the cost per reportable.

This can be a significant cost difference when determining the *total cost per year*. So, the proposal should also include the following costs: reagents, diluents, reagent grade water, calibrators, controls, consumables, and the annual maintenance fee. Usually all new instruments have a one-year warranty covering the maintenance, but years two—five will have a hefty maintenance fee, usually several thousand dollars. In addition, there may be a customer support fee, especially if the instrument has a computer monitor that can be supported via off-site interventions by tech support, when problems arise.

CHAPTER 8

Job Descriptions

In order to determine who is qualified to fill the roles of laboratory director, clinical consultant, and testing personnel, each candidate will need to know their job description as stated in the CLIA regulations. It is important to note that, as the consultant, you may need to serve in two roles. If doctors or providers cannot meet the requirements for laboratory director, the technical consultant is qualified to act as the director of a non-waived, moderate complexity lab.

Laboratory Director

The laboratory director is responsible for all aspects of laboratory operations, including, but not limited to personnel, facilities, and testing as stated in Regulation 493.1497.

§493.1407 Standard; Laboratory Director Responsibilities

The laboratory director is responsible for the overall operation and administration of the laboratory, including the employment of personnel who are competent to perform test procedures, and record and report test results promptly, accurately, and proficiently and for assuring compliance with the applicable regulations.

The laboratory director, if qualified, may perform the duties of the technical consultant, clinical consultant, and testing personnel or delegate these responsibilities to personnel meeting the qualifications of §493.1409, §493.1415, and §493.1421, respectively.

If the laboratory director reapportions performance of his or her responsibilities, he or she remains responsible for ensuring that all duties are properly performed.

The laboratory director must be accessible to the laboratory to provide onsite, telephone, or electronic consultation as needed.

Each individual may direct no more than five laboratories.

The laboratory director must:

Ensure that testing systems developed and used for each of the tests performed in the laboratory provide quality laboratory services for all aspects of test performance, which includes the pre-analytic, analytic, and post analytic phases of testing;

Ensure that the physical plant and environmental conditions of the laboratory are appropriate for the testing performed and provide a safe environment in which employees are protected for physical, chemical, and biological hazards;

Ensure that:

a. The test methodologies selected have the capability of providing the quality of results required for patient care; Verification procedures used are adequate to determine the accuracy, precision, and other pertinent performance characteristics of the method; and laboratory personnel are performing the test methods as required for accurate and reliable results;

Ensure that the laboratory is enrolled in HHS-approved proficiency testing program for the testing performed and that:

a. The proficiency testing samples are tested as required under subpart H of this part i.e. the same as patient samples

b. The results are returned within the time frames established by the proficiency-testing program.

c. All proficiency testing reports received are reviewed by the appropriate staff to evaluate the laboratory's performance and to identify any problems that require corrective action; and

d. An approved corrective action plan is followed when any proficiency testing results are found to be unacceptable or unsatisfactory.

Ensure that the quality control and quality assurance programs are established and maintained to assure the quality of laboratory services provided and to identify failures in quality as they occur.

Ensure the establishment and maintenance of acceptable levels of analytical performance for each test system.

Ensure that all necessary remedial actions are taken and documented whenever significant deviations from laboratory's established performance specifications are identified, and that patient test results are reported only when the system is functioning properly.

Ensure that reports of test results include pertinent information required for interpretation.

Ensure that consultation is available to the laboratory's clients on matters relating to the quality of the test results reported and their interpretation concerning specific patient conditions.

Employ a sufficient number of laboratory personnel with the appropriate education and either experience or training to provide appropriate consultation, properly supervise and accurately perform tests and report test results in accordance with the personnel responsibilities described.

Ensure that prior to testing patients' specimens, all personnel have the appropriate education and experience, receive the appropriate training for the type and complexity of the services offered and have demonstrated that they can accurately perform all testing operations.

Ensure that policies and procedures are established for monitoring individuals who conduct pre-analytical, analytical and post analytical phases of testing to assure that they are competent and maintain their competency to process specimens, perform test procedures and report test results promptly and proficiently, and whenever necessary, identify needs for remedial training or continuing education to improve skills.

Ensure that an approved procedure manual is available to all personnel responsible for any aspect of the testing process; and

Specify, in writing, the responsibilities and duties of each consultant and each person, engaged in the performance of the pre-analytic, analytic, and post analytic phases of testing, that identifies which examinations and procedures each individual is authorized to perform, whether supervision is required for specimen processing, test performance or results reporting, and whether consultant or director review is required prior to reporting patient test results.

Clinical Consultant

The Clinical Consultant is responsible for the clinical aspects of the laboratory operation, including, but not limited to, overseeing the requisitioning of tests, determining the medical appropriateness of the tests, and the adequacy and accuracy of test reporting as stated in Regulation 493.1457.

§493.1457 Standard; Clinical Consultant Responsibilities
    The Clinical Consultant provides consultation regarding the appropriateness of the testing ordered and interpretation of test results. The clinical consultant must:
    a. Be available to provide clinical consultation to the laboratory's clients.
    b. Be available to assist the laboratory's clients in ensuring that appropriate tests are ordered to meet the clinical expectations.
    c. Ensure that reports of test results include pertinent information required for specific patient interpretation.
    d. Ensure that consultation is available and communicated to the laboratory's clients on matters related to the quality of the test results reported and their interpretation concerning specific patient conditions.

Testing Personnel

Testing personnel are responsible for all aspects of test performance, including, but not limited to, pre-analytical, analytical, and post analytical phases of testing as stated in Regulation 493.1425.

§493.1425 Moderate or §493.1495 High Standard; Testing Personnel Responsibilities

The testing personnel are responsible for specimen processing, test performance, and for reporting test results.

Each individual performs only those moderate or high-complexity tests that are authorized by the laboratory director and require a degree of skill commensurate with the individual's education, training or experience, and technical abilities.

Each individual performing moderate complexity testing must:

Follow the laboratory's procedures for specimen handling and processing, test analysis, reporting and maintaining records of patient test results;

Maintain records that demonstrate that proficiency testing samples are tested in the same manner as patient samples;

Adhere to the laboratory's quality control policies, document all quality control activities, instrument and procedural calibrations and maintenance performed;

Follow the laboratory's established corrective action policies and procedures whenever test systems are not within the laboratory's established acceptable levels of performance;

Be capable of identifying problems that may adversely affect test performance or reporting of test results and either must correct the problems or immediately notify the technical consultant, clinical consultant or director; and

Document all corrective action taken when test systems deviate from the laboratory's established performance specifications.

If qualified under §493.1489(b)(4), must perform high complexity testing only under the onsite, direct supervision of a general supervisor qualified under §493.1461.

CHAPTER 9

Initiation of a Clinical Laboratory

Once feasibility for starting an in-house laboratory has been determined, you should establish test menu and necessary instrumentation, determine who was selected to be the laboratory director, and check to make sure the candidate is qualified. Next, look at the testing staff. Will the testing person be hired or will someone on staff do the testing?

When the doctors have named a qualified laboratory director (and it may be you) and you know the name(s) of the testing personnel and the instrument(s) needed to do the testing, you can complete the application form CMS-116 and laboratory personnel form CMS-209, both of which can be found on the CMS website (cms.gov/clia). Form CMS-116 can be found by clicking on, "How to apply for a CLIA Certificate . . . " This form is a PDF file that can be completed online and then printed, but it cannot be saved to your computer. You can find form CMS-209 on the CMS website, using the "search" function, and then print and complete it by hand. Instructions are included for completing both forms. When the forms are completed and printed, the laboratory director must sign and date them. They may be faxed or mailed to the address of the appropriate local state agency. Make sure you keep copies of each form for the laboratory's permanent records.

Processing the application may take up to three weeks, or more. Once the application is received and approved, the process moves from the state agency to central CMS billing where the bill for the CLIA license is generated and mailed to the lab for payment. Inform the accounts payable person to expect this bill and that paying the bill promptly is critical in order to keep the laboratory start-up process moving. It is important to note that *no patient testing can be started until the payment is received and posted by CMS.* If patient testing is initiated before the payment has been received and posted, any insurance claims submitted for payment prior to the receipt of the CLIA fee will likely be denied.

All medical practices order their equipment and supplies from a medical supply company. As mentioned earlier, their sales representatives can assist the practice in acquiring instrumentation, reagents, test kits, and general lab supplies, just as they do in hospitals. However, in a POL, the lab staff usually interacts with these representatives one on one. There is no purchasing department that orders reagents and supplies for the lab. Some sales representatives are knowledgeable about laboratory equipment and the proper way to put a proposal together, but others are not. It is helpful to work with knowledgeable sales representatives who can assist you in choosing the right instrumentation and supplies for the new lab. The medical practice you work with will have, in all likelihood, a sales representative who works with them for the purchase of goods and supplies. What follows is a list of just a few of the medical supply companies that regularly call on physicians' offices.

- McKesson/PSS World Medical
- Laboratory Specialists International (LSI)
- Henry Schein/MLS (Medical Laboratory Supply)
- Cardinal Health
- Fisher Scientific

One final caution, in almost every situation, once a practice has committed to starting an in-house lab, they will want it operational *yesterday*! So when you talk to the decision makers, remind them that once they commit to moving forward with this venture, it could take at least a month or two *before they start any patient testing*. It could even take longer, depending upon the kind of instrumentation required and what staff needs to be hired or trained.

Laboratory Information Systems

Computer technology has made it possible to save an immeasurable amount of time in performing the daily tasks involved in operating a laboratory. So many of the time-consuming tasks can be just a keystroke or two away from completion. There are several systems available, so be sure to contact sales representatives from several laboratory information system (LIS) companies to show you and the lab staff their product for evaluation. This is just as important as selecting the right instrument to perform patient testing.

The LIS is to the laboratory what the brain is to the human body. It can send and receive information to every part of the lab as well as to and from a patient's electronic health record (EHR). This minimizes laboratory errors, as there are no transcription errors if the results are sent electronically from the analyzer to the LIS. The LIS can be interfaced to each instrument as a unidirectional, bidirectional, or host query communication system.

Smaller instruments probably will have a unidirectional communication with the LIS, which means that it sends information to the LIS, but not the other way around. For example, a microalbumin test can be ordered on the microalbumin instrument and after running the test, the instrument will send the result back to the appropriate file in the LIS.

Bidirectional communication with the LIS means information can be sent or received by either the LIS or an instrument. For example, a chemistry panel can be ordered in the LIS and the order information then uploaded to the analyzer so that tests don't need to be ordered at the analyzer. When testing is complete, the results are transmitted back to the LIS, reviewed by the LIS, and accepted by the testing person. It is understandable that a bidirectional interface is more expensive to install than a unidirectional interface.

The host query interface has the ability to read barcodes that are generated by the LIS. The testing doesn't require uploading to the analyzer at the LIS. The analyzer is able to query the LIS based on the order/accession number and determine which tests need to be run.

The LIS can also be electronically linked to reference laboratories. When tests need to be sent to reference laboratories, the orders are created in the LIS and sent electronically to the reference lab. A manifest list of send-out tests is printed for the pick-up courier who then correlates the list against the specimens to be picked up and transported to the reference laboratory. Once the tests are completed, the results are electronically transmitted directly back to the LIS. Medical practices that have implemented an EHR and are able to incorporate the laboratory test results into the EHR as structured data. This is typically completed via an HL7 interface between the LIS and EHR. Once again, this minimizes transcription errors and saves staff time if results are currently being scanned into the health record. Providers also have the ability to order lab testing at the EHR. The orders are sent to the LIS electronically, saving the lab from manually entering the order at the LIS.

There are several tools in the LIS to assist the laboratory with ensuring that reimbursements are timely and accurate. The integration with a billing system will ensure that all laboratory charges are captured and billed. Medical necessity checking will automatically confirm that the diagnoses are appropriate for the tests ordered. This includes printing an Advanced Beneficiary Notice (ABN) for the patient to sign, stating that they are responsible for payment of the test if the testing is not covered by their insurance.

One of the most important aspects of the LIS is the link to the practice's billing department. Test "routing rules" ensure that the tests are routed to the appropriate reference laboratory so that the in-house laboratory does not perform tests for which they will not be reimbursed. There are even rules that will alert the lab about frequency of test ordering. For example, if the practitioner orders a test that the insurance company will only pay for every year and that test is ordered again within that time period, the LIS will alert the lab that this test has failed the frequency limit of the rule. This keeps the billing department from getting a denial for payment on that test and the practice will ultimately "eat the cost" of that test.

Laboratory personnel will also find that the LIS provides functionality to assist in supporting HIPPA and CLIA compliance. LIS systems will store years of QC and patient data that is readily accessible during an inspection. All corrective actions can be electronically documented and stored in the system. Many LIS systems will alert users when QC has not been run or is not within an acceptable range, when reviewing patient results. Some systems can even disallow the acceptance of results if QC has not been performed.

Storing documents electronically eliminates the need for keeping hard copies of all the information, whether it is patient results, QC, or maintenance logs, all of which were previously printed, saved and stored for two years. Note that information in an LIS should be manually or automatically backed up at least daily, on a regular basis. For laboratories with several instruments and a large test menu, a LIS is a "must have" based on the proven benefits of system integrations, increased reimbursements, and assistance with quality assurance programs.

CHAPTER 10

Selecting the Physical Location of the Laboratory

All instruments have a minimum space requirement. Become familiar with the instrument dimensions and manufacturer's recommended airflow space around the instrument. Then look at the area that has been chosen for the lab. Measure to be sure each piece of equipment will fit, especially if it will go on a counter under a cabinet.

Often an exam room is selected because it already has a sink and a small countertop. If an exam room isn't a viable option, choose an area where traffic flow is minimal. Proximity to the phlebotomy area is a plus. Other factors, such as sufficient lighting, ample electrical outlets for instruments, and a refrigerator for reagents, should be considered. One issue that often gets overlooked when deciding where to locate the lab is the heating and air conditioning supply to the lab. Since lab equipment and refrigerators generate so much heat, the lab area will require cooler room temperatures to offset this. This could be a problem if the air conditioning ducts that supply the lab with cool air are the same air conditioning ducts that supply cool air to other work areas, patient areas, or the waiting room. I have had more than one practice administrator tell me that patient's have complained about waiting rooms or exam rooms being "freezing." If the same ducts are shared between the lab and other rooms, some vents may have to be modified to balance the airflow. If this can't be done, then it might be necessary to purchase a portable air conditioner for the lab to keep the lab's room temperature within acceptable range and to keep other working areas from being too cold when the thermostat is lowered by lab staff. Remember, the comfort of lab staff is not the reason for the cool air. The technical consultant should read the manufacturer's instructions or the reagent package inserts to find information on the optimum room temperature range recommended by the manufacturer for testing samples. If you call the manufacturer's technical support line with a complaint about test result failures, they will probably ask you to fax them a history of the room temperatures. If the room temperatures are erratic or have been set out of the manufacturer's optimum range, they will not, in all likelihood, take responsibility for any test or QC failures. Whether the area designated to be the laboratory is being built or an existing area is being remodeled, I usually suggest that the lab should have separate ducts and a room temperature thermostat.

CHAPTER 11

Typical Analyzers for Various Practices

The types of tests ordered will vary depending on the specialty of the medical practice. The following are some examples of the types of medical practices, the tests they order frequently, and the types of instruments they usually have in their labs. These practices will also perform some waived testing, such as pro-thrombin time, hemoglobin A1C, urinalysis, occult blood, strep screen, and others.

General Practitioner or Family Practice Offices

The labs in these practices might resemble small hospital laboratories. They will benefit from basic chemistry and hematology analyzers. They also will perform some manual tests that are non-waived.

Countertop chemistry analyzers can perform comprehensive metabolic panels (CMP), basic metabolic panels (BMP), liver panels (LP), cardiac panels (CP), or perhaps other screening chemistry panels. These analyzers may have an assortment of several other test options that are ordered by doctors and providers, perhaps amylase or serum iron.

Unlike floor model chemistry analyzers, countertop analyzers usually require frequent calibration for each analyte. Oftentimes, the electrolytes are calibrated every eight hours. Other analytes will have their own calibration frequency. Calibrations require more hands-on time and attention by the testing person. Daily start-up and maintenance also requires more operator time and attention to perform than is required by a more sophisticated floor model type chemistry analyzer.

Countertop analyzers are initially chosen because they cost less—have a lower monthly payment—and, as the name suggests, they can fit on top of a counter, which means a smaller area is needed for the lab. The downside to countertop analyzers, aside from the more frequent calibration, is the cost per test that can be considerably more than the cost per test for a larger floor-type analyzer and slower through-put (less tests per hour). However, for smaller practices, it's sometimes a good idea to start out with a small hematology analyzer and a countertop chemistry analyzer because of the lower cost of the analyzer. Once the practice has grown and the term of the lease has expired, an upgrade to an advanced floor model chemistry analyzer and perhaps an immunology analyzer would then make more sense. (Immunology analyzers can also be countertop or floor model analyzers.)

Floor model analyzers are initially chosen because of the lower cost per test, the more extensive test menu, the faster throughput (more tests per hour), and the less hands-on operator involvement. A testing person literally puts test specimens on the instrument and can then walk away. This, however, is offset by the larger price tag of the floor analyzer itself, resulting in higher monthly lease payments.

Hematology analyzers for this type of laboratory generally fall into only one category—CBC with a three-part differential. The instruments are quite compact and take up very little room on a counter. A nearby sink is a good idea, if possible, for waste disposal. If not, a waste container can be used and routinely emptied.

Other routine non-waived tests that are ordered may include: microalbumin, mono, allergy and microscopic urine, KOH prep or wet prep. For these last four tests, I would advise against allowing them to be performed by a MA (or other unskilled testing person).

Internal Medicine Practices

These practices are similar to general practitioner and family practices in that the doctors and practitioners typically order the same kinds of chemistry and hematology tests. However, depending on the size of the practice and/or the number of practitioners, they may also order more specialized immunology tests such as thyroid panels, hormone levels, PSAs, and vitamin D and vitamin B12 tests. These tests would require an immunology analyzer for which the choices are similar to chemistry analyzers—countertop and floor models. Again, this means lower cost of analyzer for countertop models and lower cost per test for larger floor models. Here, too, test volumes are usually the determining factors. For smaller practices, it's sometimes a good idea to start out with just a hematology analyzer and countertop chemistry analyzer and then, once the practice has grown and/or the term of the lease has expired, upgrade to an advanced floor-type instrument and perhaps add an immunology analyzer.

Pain Management Practices

These practices may be part of another practice or they may be solely for the purpose of confirming the presence or absence of a drug or drugs. In either case, the instrument called for is one that can test for a myriad of drugs or drugs of abuse (DOA). Their main purpose is to confirm that a patient, who has been put on prescription drug therapy, is indeed, taking the drug. When patients complain of high levels of pain or they have had a painful surgical procedure a doctor will prescribe a drug to relieve the pain. If the patient does not take the pain medication, but instead sells the drugs to a third party the prescribing physician could get entangled in a legal situation. So, proving that the patient has taken the drug by testing urine is a must. A positive drug result proves that they have taken the drug; a negative result proves that they may not have taken the drug. A quantitative drug test is then ordered for confirmation on the same specimen. Since reagents for drug analyzer tests are very expensive, the usual procedure is to perform a drug screen, which tests for several drugs at the same time, and then perform a quantitative test for a specific drug, or drugs, for confirmation. There are a few countertop analyzers to choose from that will test for opiates, cannabinoids (THC), amphetamines, barbiturates, cocaine, ecstasy, and methadone. Some drug testing labs are high complexity and use very sophisticated instrumentation, such as mass spectrophotometry to confirm the presence of a drug. High complexity drug testing instruments can break a drug family down into specific drug subgroups or metabolites. These labs often do the drug testing for workers' compensation claims or other accident cases.

OBGYN Practices

Aside from a few waived tests, like pregnancy and urinalysis, the only laboratory tests these practices perform are for the presence of Candida, Gardnerella, and Trichomonas. Currently this tri-screen test is only performed on one instrument that I know of, manufactured by Becton Dickenson, but there may be other analyzers available as well. Often, doctors and practitioners in an OBGYN office will also perform a microscopic fern test on amniotic fluid, or wet prep and KOH prep on vaginal fluid. That is usually the extent of their laboratory test menu.

Oncology Practices

Since chemotherapy is often administered on-site at oncology practices, it is imperative that they have a hematology analyzer to perform the patient's CBC before they can administer the IV chemotherapy. Often the practice will have one or two satellite office locations that require their own CBC analyzers. Also, it is important to remember that *each geographical location must have its own CLIA license*. As these practices grow, they may decide to have one of their office laboratories become their central laboratory. Not only would the central laboratory perform its own CBC testing, but it would also perform *the entire* chemistry and tumor marker testing for the other offices as well. Patient specimens would be drawn at the other locations and couriered to the central laboratory. This actually works out very well. The serum samples can be transported to the central testing lab each day the blood is drawn or even the next day. Tumor marker tests such as PSA, CEA, CA-125, CA-27.29 or CA-15.3 are usually performed on immunology analyzers, either countertop or larger floor models.

Pediatric Practices

The only pediatric practice for which I have served as the technical consultant has two identical CBC analyzers, one for the "sick child side," and one for the "well child side." The analyzers they use are well suited for this type of practice because the blood specimen is collected in a capillary tube, thereby avoiding a traumatic venipuncture for the child.

The pediatric practice also performs a confirmation culture on all negative Streptococcus screens. By performing a confirmatory culture, they are able to catch those early infections that may give a negative screening test but, in fact, grow the Streptococcus organism, resulting in a positive throat culture for Streptococcus. The only instrument required is a small 37° incubator. The doctor or provider collects two throat swabs. One swab is used for the Streptococcus screen; the other is inoculated onto a blood agar (BA) plate and streaked for isolation. A bacitracin or Taxo A disc is placed on the primary inoculation area. The plate is then incubated for twenty-four hours for initial reading of beta hemolysis using the bacitracin or Taxo A disc to indicate growth resistance, the presumptive presence of Streptococcus Group A. The final culture reading is taken forty-eight hours after inoculation.

Specialty Practices

It has been my experience that specialty practices like endocrinology and cardiology often do not have in-house labs, but if they do, they are best served by a routine chemistry analyzer and/or an immunology analyzer.

It is important to note that insurance carriers will only allow a set number of test panels or individual tests to be performed on a patient *within a specific time period*. For example, allergy panels may only be performed on a patient once per year. Exceptions may apply for various diagnoses or for abnormal test results. Repeat testing of a test panel or individual tests may result in denial of an insurance claim.

Accountable Care Organizations

To counteract some of the rising Medicare costs, the new Obama-Care allows for larger groups of doctors to form an accountable care organization or ACO. According to CMS, an ACO is "an organization of health care providers that agrees to be accountable for the quality, cost and overall care of Medicare beneficiaries who are enrolled in the traditional fee-for-service program who are assigned to it." In other words, these organizations are made up of a large group of doctors, possibly several hundred doctors and providers. Each may have his/her own general or specialty practice, but unite to start up one large laboratory or "medical mall." Laboratory testing that is performed on their collective patients can reduce the unnecessary duplication of lab tests that would otherwise happen if the tests were ordered by multiple health care providers on the same patient and unite smaller practices that otherwise would be too small to have an in-house lab of their own. Laboratory tests and equipment could include all of the instrumentation afore-mentioned.

CHAPTER 12

What Is an Instrument Reagent Rental?

Some instrument manufacturers will offer something called a reagent rental in lieu of an instrument purchase or instrument lease. This has been a popular option when choosing which instrument the lab will use to perform their testing.

This is how it works. The estimated test volumes for each test that can be performed on a new instrument are determined. Based on the *estimated* test volumes, the monthly amount of reagents or reagent kits is then determined. A contract between the medical practice and the instrument manufacturer is created that states the minimum number of test reagents or reagent kits the medical practice agrees to purchase *every* month for the term of the contract. A new instrument is provided free of charge and installed for the laboratory to use for their testing without paying a monthly cost for the instrument or instrument maintenance fees. Sound enticing?

Here's the downside. Instrument shipping fees for the instrument could be the responsibility of the medical practice and can be expensive. Also, remember that the number of reagents or reagent kits will be based on an *estimated* number of monthly tests. So, if the practice doesn't use the minimum number of reagents or reagent kits each month, guess what? The lab will be required to pay the monthly rental fee and will also continue to receive their minimum shipment of reagents or reagent kits each month. This will be stated in the agreement. I have seen labs stockpile reagents that they didn't use because their estimated

36

test volumes weren't correct. They hoped they could stay ahead of the expiration dates until their test volumes went up. So, be reasonably sure the test volume estimates are accurate, even if that means underestimating monthly test volumes. After all, the rental agreement should not contain wording that says you cannot purchase *more* than the number of reagents or kits per month. Lastly, I have observed one manufacturer that provided an instrument for reagent rental, phased it out, and then no longer supported the instrument's testing, which is to say the lab would no longer be able to buy any reagents, calibrators, supplies, or receive maintenance and service. The manufacturer could then promote their upgraded instrument whose test menu included the SAME TESTS as offered by their previous instrument plus some additional tests which, in my experience, were too specialized and would not be utilized by a POL. The new instrument also required a new reagent rental agreement and the instrument had to be shipped, installed, and validated. It required new reagents, calibrators, and supplies leaving any leftover reagents, calibrators or supplies from the discontinued instrument to be thrown out!

CHAPTER 13

Personnel Hiring and Training

Hiring

Gone are the days of placing an expensive ad in the newspaper for laboratory positions. Today, someone searching for a new job does an Internet search on such sites as Indeed.com, which can connect them to various job websites for clinical laboratory positions. If a practice does not have a qualified staff member or someone else that could be trained to perform lab testing, then posting the position online is a good start. If the new laboratory will have several lab instruments, the testing person should have previous experience working in a lab or have had laboratory education and training. If the person hired has *no* lab experience and is not familiar with daily tasks such as QC, QA, proficiency testing, or maintenance, this could lead to poor work performance and a headache for you and the practice. Often the doctors or administrators think they can pay a lower wage to an inexperienced testing person . . . big mistake. They don't realize how expensive testing reagents can be; therefore, their misuse due to handling by inexperienced personnel can cost them more in the long run than paying a higher wage to a knowledgeable and trained individual.

If the ad is placed on a website, the technical consultant may want to be assistive in writing the ad to avoid getting ill-suited applicants. I would suggest incorporating statements in the ad, such as, "Prefer experience in operating the following equipment . . ." or, "Knowledge of hematology and chemistry analyzers a plus." These statements will help to weed out inexperienced and unskilled applicants. Request the applicants to send a resume for review.

After several resumes have been received, the technical consultant should review these and choose the best three applicants for the practice administrator to interview. That way you have some control over the initial screening of applicants, and the hiring process can begin. Applicants who have the most experience with similar lab instruments or have other lab skills should be interviewed first. If none of the applicants has had experience operating lab instruments similar to those in the new lab, then applicants with other lab skills should be considered. It will be up to the practice administrator to conduct the personal interviews with the initial candidates you've screened and to evaluate other qualifications and qualities that are a good fit for the practice.

Training

For simple-to-run analyzers, most manufacturers have field staff who will come to the lab and train the testing personnel on-site. After training is complete, training certificates are typically awarded. The technical consultant should follow up with trained personnel to ensure that training certificates get put into personnel files. The original trainee(s) can then train future testing personnel and a training document can be created and placed in the personnel file of the new trainee.

For more complex analyzers or multiple analyzers, most manufacturers will train one staff person at an off-site training facility. Travel expenses, meals, and lodging are arranged and usually paid for by the manufacturer. Training can take up to a week for chemistry and immunology analyzers. That means an employee will be away from their duties at the practice during that time. Often, the new analyzer will be installed and validated, while the lab employee is at training. Installations by service technicians can also take several days.

It is the laboratory's obligation to ensure compliance with CLIA regulations for precision, linearity, calibration, and QC validation studies on any new instrument. Most instrument service technicians, as a courtesy, will perform and document most, it not all, of these studies. It is up to the technical consultant, or lab director, to review and accept these studies and sign off on them. If a service technician does not complete all of these studies, it is the responsibility of the testing personnel to perform them.

Once completed, an accuracy check on the new analyzer must be performed. The purpose of this is to compare the accuracy of the test results from the new analyzer with the manufacturer's accuracy assertions. To check the accuracy of the instrument, I recommend commercially available materials, calibrators, and QC or proficiency samples. All of these have known values that can be used to compare the accuracy assertion. If results of the testing fall within the acceptable limits of the material used, then the accuracy check passes. Another way to perform an accuracy check is to send half of a serum sample to a reference lab to perform the tests that will be performed in-house and run the same tests on the other half on the new analyzer. Results should compare closely with one another. I usually suggest they compare within two standard deviations. Although CLIA regulations don't state exactly how many samples must be compared, twenty samples is good lab practice. The only time I might recommend less than twenty samples is if the test is very expensive to run. In that case, ten samples may be acceptable to your COLA or CLIA inspector. Once the accuracy check is completed, results may be reviewed and accepted by the technical consultant or laboratory director. Only then can patient testing begin.

It is the technical consultant's responsibility to be involved with non-instrument training: going over any forms that need to be completed or recording pertinent data. The manufacturer should provide these forms, which should include maintenance logs, reagent logs, QC logs, calibration logs, temperature logs, and any other record-keeping documents that require ongoing documentation as a result of operating the new analyzer.

The technical consultant can recommend to testing personnel that it is advisable to request the same lot number when ordering several boxes of the same reagent or kit. Doing this may reduce the need to recalibrate a new lot number and rerun QC again.

One of the most important things a technical consultant can do to encourage new laboratory staff is to emphasize the importance of the testing person's job to help them realize what a special role they play in the patient-care process. They need to be reminded that each test they perform and report to the doctor is an important piece of information that directly affects a patient's diagnosis and/or treatment.

Training lab staff is an ongoing process. For each laboratory on which you consult, you should schedule regular on-site visits to monitor the endless list of tasks and to establish a good working relationship with the staff. In addition, you must be available by e-mail and phone during business hours to answer questions, give advice, or help with problem solving. Respond to all voicemails, texts, and e-mails promptly. The quicker your response, the faster you can answer questions or assist in problem resolution.

CHAPTER 14

On-site Consulting Visits

Regular monthly or bimonthly visits to the practice are the best way to establish strong relationships with laboratory and administrative staff and doctors. Especially the lab staff, since there usually isn't any other "go to" person in the practice to help them with day-to-day lab issues that frequently arise. Unless you visit each lab on a regular basis, it will be more difficult to establish a camaraderie and loyalty with the lab staff. The last thing I want to hear as a consultant is that problems couldn't be resolved in a timely manner because I wasn't readily available to the lab staff and they had to fend for themselves.

It is my strong belief that the technical consultant should visit small labs, those with only one instrument and a few manual tests, once a month. Larger labs—ones with a hematology analyzer, chemistry analyzer, one or more instruments, and those doing several manual tests—should be visited twice per month. I suggest you visit during the first week of each month for every lab. This will give you the opportunity to review the QC, maintenance logs, temperature logs, proficiency evaluations, calibrations, and other monthly records that the lab has recorded for the previous month. It is your responsibility to review and sign off on each of these records. This regular practice will keep you current with quality assurance reviews and also give you the opportunity to communicate with lab staff, doctors, practitioners, administrators, and ancillary office staff. At the end of your visit, you can be assured that everything is organized and records and documentation are properly filed and stored.

If you detect a problem during your visits or have questions as a result of reviewing records, you can address them on the spot. In the end, you will find great satisfaction in working hand-in-hand with laboratory staff and serving as a touchstone for questions and concerns. You and the laboratory staff will be working as a team to achieve the goal of CLIA compliance, good patient care, and laboratory profitability,

It is important that you do not let more than a month or two to pass before reviewing QC documents and addressing quality assessment issues. If you fail to do this, you may discover a problem that is too far downstream to correct easily, if at all, stressing the need for regular on-site visits. Each visit to a lab will solidify your standing with the practice and demonstrate your dedication to helping and supporting the lab staff. *You* are their lifeline, their answer person, and their problem solver. The lab staff, in turn, will support you when the inevitable question is asked, "What does the technical consultant do, anyway?"

It is advisable that you maintain a consistent interaction with not only the laboratory staff, but also the entire office staff. Oftentimes, other staff members feel inept when lab-related problems arise. Make them feel comfortable enough to pick up the phone or send you an e-mail if they need your help. Remembering the names of staff members and calling them by name will establish a bond with them. They say that the sweetest sound in any language is the sound of a person's name. Try it.

Every week I create a schedule for lab visits that I can print and take with me to review as I travel from office to office. When I'm finished with a visit, I write a synopsis of the visit, or just note a comment on my schedule. When the week is over, I file the schedule and keep it for future reference.

For more complex labs with larger test menus and instrumentation, it is advisable to have monthly meetings with lab staff, the laboratory director, and any administrative personnel who are involved with the lab. It is helpful to have one of the lab staff prepare an agenda and send it out a few days ahead of time to attendees. QA issues or problems that have come up recently can be addressed and acted upon. Future agendas can address and review the follow-up actions to these issues.

CHAPTER 15

Off-site Consulting

While off-site consulting would not be my preference, I realize that there are some circumstances in which a technical consultant has no choice but to consult for a laboratory that is located at a distance. Because I have been lucky enough to work in Phoenix and surrounding areas, I have not had to drive so far away that I could not visit labs on a regular basis. Having said that, I recognize that in sparsely populated areas or in small cities, there may be no choice other than an off-site consulting arrangement. QC and calibration documentation, maintenance logs, and anything in hard copy can be mailed, faxed or e-mailed as an attachment to the consultant for review. In the future, these documents will likely be available through secured "cloud" storage. Phone communication, e-mail, and texting are all possible means of communicating with lab staff or doctors in an effort to maintain and keep laboratories in compliance with CLIA regulations. In such cases, consultants will make an on-site visit every three or four months and spend the better part of the day tending to those duties that can only be accomplished on-site.

So, although this is not the ideal way to provide technical consulting for a laboratory, it is the only way to provide technical consulting in those situations where the lab is geographically just too far away to provide frequent or regular on-site laboratory visits.

CHAPTER 16

Overseeing Unskilled Lab Staff—Medical Assistants

An unfortunate outcome of the Clinical Laboratory Improvement Amendments of 1988 was to allow people with only high school diplomas or GEDs to perform non-waived (moderately complex), clinical laboratory testing. Medical technologists with four years of higher education and a bachelor's degree in science are often appalled at that notion. However, technology has made many instruments easier to operate when performing testing and several have advanced governing systems that prevent patient testing when QC fails, a lot number has expired, or calibration is due. For almost all point-of-care analyzers, the manufacturer provides field staff that will train one or more unskilled testing personnel. Often they may spend several hours training the new medical assistant (MA) as well as qualified testing personnel. It is advisable to train more than one staff member since the primary testing person, or MA, may call in sick or even leave the practice, creating a situation where another trainee must step in to perform testing.

Monitoring the work of new testing staff is an ongoing task for the technical consultant. As an educated and experienced laboratorian, the technical consultant will find it impossible to know the skill level of the MA. Your head is filled with years of experience and knowledge that you simply can't expect them to know. In addition to knowledge and experience, some testing personnel may not be adept in organizational skills, mechanical skills, logic, or common sense. Recognizing which of these skills a MA possesses, or doesn't possess, is important so that you can help him/her to improve those skills. It is also advisable to compliment them when they improve.

One of the biggest concerns with MAs is that they often are short-term employees. Many times they leave suddenly or give little notice. The revolving door situation associated with MA staff makes it difficult to run a lab smoothly if they are performing primary testing. When a MA leaves the practice, another testing person can be assigned the testing responsibilities from the group of other MAs or staff who attended the initial training. If there is a backup testing person already in place, that is a big help. The technical consultant should reinforce the importance of the duties he/she performs, which will help to retain the MA as a stable laboratory employee.

CHAPTER 17

Overseeing Skilled Lab Staff—MLTs or CLAs

New testing personnel with a diploma from an accredited MLT or CLA program will have at least a basic knowledge of how a lab functions. It's a bonus if they have previously worked in a POL, so they can provide assistance in transitioning into the new laboratory. However, every lab is different—resulting in different experiences—so guidance from a technical consultant is always necessary. Initially, frequent visits by the technical consultant may be necessary. The training and experience MLTs and CLAs received in school in performing testing on various instruments is often learned on analyzers they won't ever see again. Their knowledge and education may be useful, but their *experience* with several different instruments may be limited.

There never seems to be an end to questions or problem situations in the clinical lab. One of the biggest challenges for a MLT or CLA is to learn how to use the LIS. Every system has its own unique operating system and it may take several weeks for a new employee to feel confident in using one. Additionally, the medical practice's EHR is another learning hurdle that will take time to learn.

The technical consultant's questions during visits often uncover seemingly minor concerns for the MLT or CLA, but can be just the tip of the iceberg of a problem, one that could become much larger. For example, I remember the time I went into a lab for a visit and found out they had *not* printed background counts from their hematology instrument for several days. When I asked why, I was told that the printer was out of ink! Fortunately, during that visit we were able to access the missing background counts in the analyzer's data log and print the saved records. If this had not been corrected, their next inspection would have been in jeopardy of a deficiency citation for not keeping laboratory records for two years and not having proof that the daily start-up passed. Therefore, the technical consultant's visits are the glue that holds the lab together and what keeps the required documentation up-to-date.

New laboratories performing non-waived testing that have a MLT or CLA performing the lab tests typically stand a better chance of CLIA compliance and financial success. This is because decision makers associated with the practice have committed themselves to hiring skilled lab staff, which is instrumental in making it succeed. As new providers are added to the practice and the lab test menu is expanded, more testing will be done. As test volumes increase, it may be time to add more equipment, another testing person, and possibly a MA.

At some time during this growth, it is the technical consultant's responsibility to research the tests that are *not* being tested in-house, but are instead routinely sent out to reference laboratories. It may be feasible to add these tests to the lab's existing test menu. You will need to ask several questions.

- Does the in-house lab have the capability of performing these tests?
- Are the volumes of these tests high enough?
- Will they require additional instrumentation?

If you answered yes to any of these questions, recommend to decision makers that they seriously consider adding more instrumentation and new tests to their test menu. They'll figure out on their own that more testing means more income for the practice. The side benefit to you is that this will underscore the value you bring to their practice by adding more on-site patient testing, creating faster turnaround times for results, and generating more financial gain for the practice.

CHAPTER 18

Choosing a Proficiency Testing Agency

Proficiency testing in the POL is very much the same as the proficiency testing done in a hospital's clinical laboratory. Participating in a proficiency program is critically important to the operation of the laboratory and a must for CLIA compliance.

CLIA Regulation §493.1236©(1) Evaluation Of Proficiency Testing Performance states:
At least twice annually, the laboratory must verify the accuracy of any test or procedure it performs.

Participating with an approved off-site proficiency-testing program is typically done for verifying accuracy. There are several proficiency programs that offer this accuracy check for a laboratory's non-waived (moderately complex *and* highly complex) tests. It is most important to make sure the proficiency-testing program can offer proficiency testing for *all* non-waived tests performed in the laboratory.

There are factors to consider when choosing a proficiency-testing agency, including proficiency testing fees that vary depending on which test or test groups are being ordered. You can check with several organizations before making a recommendation for selecting an agency.

Most proficiency testing agencies send test samples to the lab three times a year, commonly referred to as three "test events" per year. These are samples that the in-house lab will test in the same way they test patient specimens and then report their results to the proficiency agency where the results are scored. Some labs prefer to choose a proficiency agency that will divide the test samples into specialties and send out test samples for each specialty separately. Therefore, instead of sending the samples for chemistry, immunology, hematology, serology, and micro-biology all at one time, each specialty shipment is staggered several weeks apart. This seems to work better for larger labo-ratories with hematology, chemistry, immunology, serology, and microbiology testing specialties. This avoids work overload that happens when testing is done for all the samples at one time for every testing event.

CLIA Approved Proficiency Testing Programs 2012

Accutest, Inc.
P.O. Box 999
Westford, Massachusetts 01886
(800) 665-2575

AAFP-PT
11400 Tomahawk Creek Parkway
Leawood, Kansas 66211-2672
(800) 274-7911

American Association Of Bioanalysts (AAB)
205 West Levee Street
Brownsville, Texas 78520-5596
(800) 234-5315

American Proficiency Institute (API)
1159 Business Park Drive
Traverse City, Michigan 49686
(800) 333- 0958

California Thoracic Society (CTS)
575 Market Street
Suite 2125
San Francisco, California 94105
(415) 536-0287`

The College Of American Pathologists (CAP) Surveys
College of American Pathologists
325 Waukegan Road
Northfield, Illinois 60093-2750
(847) 832-7000

External Comparative Evaluation For Laboratories—Excel
College of American Pathologists
325 Waukegan Road
Northfield, Illinois 60093-2750
(800) 323-4040

Medical Laboratory Evaluation (MLE) Program
25 Massachusetts Avenue, NW
Suite 700
Washington, DC 20001-7401
(800) 338-2746, (202) 261-4500

Commonwealth Of Pennsylvania
Department of Health
Bureau of Laboratories
P.O. Box 500
Exton, Pennsylvania 19341-0500
(610) 280-3464

Puerto Rico Proficiency Testing Service
Public Health Laboratories of Puerto Rico
PO Box 70184
San Juan, Puerto Rico 00936-8184
(787) 274-6827

WSLH (Wisconsin State Health Lab)
Proficiency Testing Program
465 Henry Mall
Madison, Wisconsin 53706-1578
(800) 462-5261

American Society For Clinical Pathology
8900 Keystone Crossing
Suite 620
Indianapolis, IN 46240
(800) 267-2727, (317) 876-4169

New York State Department Of Health
State of New York
Department of Health
The Governor Nelson A. Rockefeller State Plaza
P.O. Box 509
Albany, New York 12201-0509
(518) 474-8739

A laboratory located outside the State of New York that holds a valid New York State permit may choose to use the New York State proficiency-testing (PT) program to fulfill federal requirements for PT enrollment and participation in the specialties of micro bacteriology, diagnostic immunology, chemistry, hematology, and immunohematology.

While there are several, the proficiency-testing agency with which I am most familiar is the American Proficiency Institute (API). I would encourage you to choose the one that best fits the lab's needs and requirements.

Some of the features I prefer in a proficiency-testing agency are as follows:

• A person answers the phone when you call

    There is no automated message that sends you through a myriad of menus as you wait and listen to music for several minutes. Speaking with someone immediately is especially helpful when lab personnel cannot proceed with testing without help or if there is a problem with submitting their results.

- Proficiency shipments are staggered

  Each shipment for chemistry, immunology, hematology, and microbiology test samples are separate shipments. As mentioned, this is particularly helpful when there is only one testing person to perform testing on all proficiency samples for all tests performed in a laboratory. Breaking it up into separate shipments with different due dates is so much better.

- E-mail alerts are sent

  The proficiency agency notifies each laboratory to tell them when the next proficiency event will be shipped: Technical consultants get e-mail notifications alerting them of labs with test failures for the last event: A failure report is attached to the e-mail, which allows the technical consultant to take immediate action to investigate the problem and determine why it occurred so that the technical consultant and lab staff can determine resolution.

- Access to the agency's website

  With access to this site, the technical consultant can see the lab's testing score histories for the laboratories with which they consult. This is extremely helpful in identifying failure trends, which may prompt you to question when an instrument was last calibrated, or if personnel need additional training to conduct testing. After reviewing failed results, you will discover that the reason for the failure may simply have been a data entry error where the results for two different samples were flip-flopped. The error could also be the result of a misplaced decimal or something transcribed incorrectly. This can easily be verified by comparing the submitted proficiency results with the lab instrument's printout or the patient log (where proficiency test sample results are recorded).

- Ability to check the proficiency's website to monitor that your labs have reported their proficiency test results before the due date

  If you see that a lab has not submitted their results and it is not past the deadline, contact the lab staff to check the status of the proficiency testing completion and remind them of the due date. I remember a few instances when a front office person put the proficiency samples in the refrigerator and lab staff was not notified. This caused needless panic and angst amongst co-workers; they ended up submitting their results *after* the due date and a self-evaluation had to be written.

- The option to obtain a report for laboratories that have not re-ordered their proficiency testing for the coming year

  Near the end of each year, it's important to obtain this report to make sure an order for proficiency testing is completed since failing to do so could result in a missed shipment for the first testing event the next year. A reorder must be placed each year. Often, this doesn't get discovered until after the first event samples in the following year have already been shipped, in which case it is too late to correct the oversight. On their next CLIA inspection, the inspector will see that you have a failure for the entire testing event. It's important when ordering or reordering proficiency testing that you make sure the proficiency agency sends a copy of each lab's scores to COLA or the state CLIA agency and also to you, the technical consultant.

- The ability to request additional proficiency samples for new tests in the next testing event when a new instrument or test is added in the laboratory

  If a new test or instrument is added and the next testing event is more than a month or two away, you should request that the agency send leftover proficiency samples for new test(s). Test results will not be evaluated and there will not be a due date. However, along with the samples, the agency will send the acceptable result ranges for the new test(s). The testing personnel can write a self-evaluation that can be reviewed by the technical consultant, or the technical consultant can write it. These samples are not free, but it is good laboratory practice and it will keep the lab CLIA compliant.

Caution: the proficiency agency may not always have any leftover samples to send you.

CHAPTER 19

Preparing for Proficiency Specimen Arrival

Request a copy of the shipping schedule from the proficiency agency and post it in the laboratory. The shipping date and due date for each specialty and each event will be on the schedule. The technical consultant should also keep a copy and maintain a master calendar to remind lab staff a week or so ahead of when proficiency samples are due to arrive. Especially in new laboratories, the front office personnel or the person who receives FedEx, UPS, or USPS (United States Postal Service) deliveries should be notified a day or two ahead in advance of when a proficiency shipment is due to arrive. In most cases, the delivery package *must be refrigerated upon arrival,* so the person taking receipt must remember to put it in a designated lab refrigerator immediately upon arrival or give it to a lab person to do that.

Shortly after the shipping date, the technical consultant should verify that the proficiency samples have been received. Remind them of the due date and check back with them if you see, via the proficiency's website, that results have not been submitted. Once a routine for the proficiency testing process has been established, future shipments and result submissions will go smoothly.

CHAPTER 20

Submitting Proficiency Test Results

After all the proficiency samples have been tested, it is important to freeze them, with the exception of whole blood samples. These saved samples can be used later to check the accuracy of a test method whenever a problem arises or can be used as training samples to check the competency of new testing personnel. They are useful because they have known values with ranges of acceptability. They can be retested and used as a comparison to validate the accuracy of a test. Often these frozen proficiency samples can be useful when investigating and solving numerous testing problems.

Read all the information contained in the proficiency instructions accompanying the samples. When testing is complete and testing personnel are ready to submit the results by mail, remember that a machine might be reading the result forms, so writing numbers or filling in bubbles must be done *exactly* as the instructions specify. Keep all numbers inside the answer box and *do not cross out or write over numbers*. This could lead to misinterpretation of the result(s) and thus a failed score. Typically, proficiency sample test results must be sent back to the proficiency agency within ten to twelve working days from the receipt date of the samples, depending on whether the results are mailed, faxed, or submitted online.

Proficiency results can be mailed, faxed, or transmitted online to the proficiency agency. I strongly recommend that results be submitted online, as this will give the lab staff, and you, peace of mind in knowing that these have been submitted and received on time. Lab staff can also print a copy of online submissions to keep for their records. If lab staff chooses to fax results, they should print a copy of the fax confirmation and keep it for their records along with all the original instrument printouts and patient result logs. If the lab staff chooses to mail in proficiency results, they must make copies of the result forms for their records and then take their submitted results to the post office *before the due date* to ensure they get postmarked in time.

If there is a problem performing testing, because the instrument is "down" or because a test reagent or kit is back ordered or because the testing personnel were unable to perform the testing, the proficiency agency should be called immediately to alert them of the problem. They will let the caller know what to do, how to communicate the problem to the proficiency agency, and advise them of the best way to document the issue to prevent a failed score.

It is good laboratory practice to have a separate file for any proficiency records in the lab. That includes copies of anything sent to the proficiency agency by fax, USPS, FedEx, UPS, or electronically. Practice administrators or human resources personnel may also want to have a copy of all proficiency documents for their records.

CHAPTER 21

Reordering
Proficiency Testing

By the end of the year, proficiency testing may not have been ordered for the following year. There can be many reasons for this, despite the fact that proficiency-testing agencies usually include a reminder with the third event's evaluation scores or send an e-mail reminder to order proficiency testing. These reminder notices should be forwarded to the accounts payable person or the practice administrator, so someone can reorder. The technical consultant should ask to see a copy of the order confirmation. If the technical consultant hasn't seen this confirmation by December, the lab may be in jeopardy of not receiving samples for the first event early enough the next year. It's important that the order confirmation include *new tests* that may have been added since the last proficiency event.

Order information for new tests can be found in the proficiency agency's catalog located on the proficiency's website or by calling their customer service department. Again, be sure the accounts payable person is aware of any changes so the proper payment can be made.

Proficiency Testing Reminders

Follow these important proficiency-testing guidelines:

* Print and post the yearly schedule of proficiency agency shipment dates and due dates.

- Test proficiency samples in exactly the same manner as patient samples.
- Ensure that patient-testing personnel have participated in proficiency testing on a rotating basis.
- Ensure that testing personnel who test proficiency samples have signed attestation statements.
- Ensure that the laboratory director or qualified designee has signed attestation statements.
- Submit all proficiency test results by the due date and time.
- If the integrity of proficiency samples is compromised in shipment, call the proficiency agency immediately to register or resolve the problem or to request new samples, and then document the date and time of the call.
- Ensure that all non-waived tests performed by the laboratory have proficiency testing performed unless a CLIA approved alternative accuracy check has been done.
- Make copies of all submitted results and comments.
- Keep all paperwork related to each testing event, including original instructions and instrument printouts in a separate proficiency testing binder and save them for two years.
- Freeze all proficiency samples when testing is complete (except whole blood samples).
- Write corrective action reports on failed proficiency scores.

CHAPTER 22

Proficiency Testing Failures

CLIA regulations require that any proficiency evaluation score of 80 percent or less be documented in a corrective action report. For all regulated analytes, the proficiency agency will send five unknown samples per test or per panel of tests. If only one of the five results per analyte submitted falls outside the range of acceptability, resulting in a score for that analyte of 80 percent, a corrective action report must be written that includes the following:

- An explanation of the problem or why you believe the result obtained was unacceptable.
- A statement of whether patient care was affected and if so, an investigation must be conducted, via chart review of patients recently tested for that test. Document the investigation and write a corrective action report.
- Based on the investigation and the corrective action report, write an explanation of whether or not this test failure has the potential to affect future patient care.
- Explain what corrective action or training was done to monitor and/or prevent the failure from happening again.
- Explain what system changes or measures have been put in place to ensure this failure won't happen again.

Asking the technical consultant to assist in documenting these requirements is advisable. The laboratory director and/ or technical consultant should review the corrective action with testing personnel and sign the report.

In almost every case if the proficiency score is 0 percent, it is due to a clerical error. One of the most common failures resulting in a score of 0 percent (especially for a new laboratory performing CBCs) is when the testing person who submits the test results reports the *actual* result for the CBC's differential instead of the *percent* values. Inexperienced testing personnel frequently get this wrong the first time they enter differential results because the CBC instrument report format usually lists differential actual values first and then percent values. The lower the score(s) are for the failed analyte(s), the bigger the problem. Once a failure of 60 percent or less is reported, the technical consultant should start an investigation to determine why the failures occurred and follow up with a corrective action report. Keep the report and all other documents pertaining to each test event for two years.

CLIA regulations state that if a proficiency test fails two out of three proficiency test events, including a failure to submit results by the due date, the lab will receive a letter from their state agency stating that the laboratory was not in compliance with the *conditions* of successful participation in proficiency testing. The letter will state that the laboratory has had an unsatisfactory performance in proficiency testing and must submit a "credible allegation of compliance and acceptable evidence of correction." In the future, if the laboratory fails proficiency testing again, the CMS regional office will become involved to initiate sanctions against the laboratory's CLIA certificate. The sanctions may include monetary penalties, suspension of Medicare payments, cancellation of Medicare payments, or revocation of the laboratory's CLIA certificate. "Condition-level deficiencies are cited when the deficient practice is so serious that corrections are necessary for the laboratory testing to continue." Laboratories that do not meet the condition-level requirement of CLIA may not be certified to perform testing and a cease-and-desist letter will follow. The laboratory will be given a due date, usually ten days from the receipt of the letter, to complete and submit the credible allegation of compliance.

A credible allegation of compliance letter is written by a representative of the laboratory who has a history of maintaining a commitment to compliance and taking the required corrective action and will include a statement that the corrective action is feasible and is being accomplished and a resolution to the problem stating the action taken as follows:

- Investigation conducted of patients affected or those who have the potential to become affected by the deficiency
- Changes that were made to ensure deficiency does not recur.
- Changes in place to continue to monitor to ensure that the failure does not recur.

Laboratory directors who find themselves in trouble with CLIA have asked me to help them resolve their conditional-level deficiencies. It should never be taken lightly how much power the government has or the penalties that they can assess. Once word has spread of sanctions levied by CLIA, it's no wonder that many doctors fear CLIA inspectors and are hesitant to have their own in-house laboratory. Technical consultants are also not surprised that so many doctors who assume the role of director *and* technical consultant end up in trouble. In my opinion, doctors should stick to what they do best . . . doctoring, and leave the ongoing technical oversight of the laboratory to an experienced technical consultant.

CHAPTER 23

CLIA Inspections 101

COLA, Inc. was founded in 1988 and was known as the Commission on Office Laboratory Assessment. COLA is an accreditation and educational alternative program for physician office laboratories and was granted that authority under CLIA by CMS in 1993. Physicians can choose between the government's program and COLA's program for their CLIA inspection service. COLA surveys and state CLIA surveys, more commonly called inspections, are scheduled every other year unless the laboratory is new.

Notice for an upcoming inspection can be sent by regular mail or by e-mail and generally arrives about two weeks before the date of the scheduled inspection. The date will be chosen based on the inspector's schedule. If the date chosen is not convenient for you or the lab staff, a change can be requested, but probably will not be rescheduled without a good reason. COLA can even charge the practice an additional fee for changing the inspection date.

CLIA inspections will most likely be conducted by an inspector from the department of health services (DHS), a.k.a. "state agency," or by COLA. All laboratories are charged an inspection fee for their initial and subsequent biennial inspections. This is a separate fee from the biennial license fee that is usually billed one year to six months before the CLIA license expires.

State Agency CLIA Inspections

The purpose of a state agency CLIA inspection is to renew the Certificate of Compliance when a successful completion of an on-site inspection for non-waived testing is conducted. For existing laboratories, the inspection is usually conducted six months prior to the date of expiration indicated on the CLIA license. The new CLIA license is mailed to the laboratory about two weeks prior to the existing expiration date on the license.

For new laboratories, the first CLIA inspection is conducted within the first year following license application and acceptance. That means the one-year clock starts ticking as soon as the CLIA license application has been accepted and the license fee has been paid. Some states may require that an initial inspection be conducted *before* patient testing commences.

Remember that starting a lab takes time. Insurance contract negotiations to accept in-house laboratory testing, test menu and LIS selection, instrument evaluations and installation, lab staff hiring, and training can take weeks or months before the lab is up and running for patient testing. When these tasks fall behind schedule, patient testing could be delayed for several weeks or even months. If this happens, you may be surprised when patient testing has just recently begun and the inspection notice arrives that your first inspection has been scheduled! I remember three situations when the laboratory received notice of the date of their first inspection and the patient testing had not yet begun. My reason for including this situation is to advise the technical consultant not to submit an application for a CLIA license or to upgrade a waived license too soon. It would be better to have the CMS-116 completed and ready to submit when the new laboratory space is ready for equipment, the test menu has been chosen, and there is an agreement on the instrument(s) needed for testing.

The letter sent to the lab announcing the date of the upcoming CLIA inspection might include a list of materials or information the inspector would like to review during the inspection.

- Policy and procedure manuals, package inserts, and safety information
- Quality assessment plan

- Quality assessment records for the past two years
- Proficiency testing records for the past two years, including report forms, attestation statements, instruments printouts, and evaluation reports from the proficiency testing agency
- Instrument maintenance records for the past two years, including installation records for instruments and service information
- Quality control records
- Personnel files, including up-to-date medical licenses, proof of education (diploma or transcript), and job descriptions for laboratory personnel, training records, and timely competency evaluations
- Patient logs, if applicable
- Copy of an in-house test order, if applicable
- Annual test volumes for each test specialty performed, including waived tests, provider performed microscopy procedures (PPMP), and their annual volumes

The notification letter should include two forms: CMS-209 and CMS-116. Form CMS-209 is the Laboratory Personnel Report (CLIA), which requires the names of all lab employees, their position(s), and their work schedules. Form CMS-116 is the same form that was used when the lab applied for a CLIA license, and the same information is typically entered again, except at the top of the first page, the "survey" box is to be checked. Both forms must be *completed and signed* by the laboratory director and returned to the inspector during the inspection entrance interview. Be sure that this is completed and signed ahead of the inspection date.

Depending on the size of the lab (number of testing personnel, test menu, number and type of instrumentation, and any deficiency problems uncovered during the inspection) an inspection can last anywhere from two to six hours. After the inspection is completed, the lab will be sent a follow-up letter from the inspector.

Cathy L. Manske

COLA Inspections

The purpose of the COLA inspection is to renew the Certificate of Accreditation following the successful completion of an on-site inspection including non-waived and waived tests.

Although most of the inspections I have been involved with were Arizona state inspections, I have had several that were conducted by COLA, whose motto is "Lab Accreditation Through Education." It should be emphasized that when a lab is affiliated with COLA for their CLIA license, the lab receives a Certificate of *Accreditation* not a Certificate of *Certification* as with state agency CLIA inspections. Wikipedia defines these two terms as follows:

- Compliance is adherence to standards, regulations, and other requirements.
- Accreditation is a process in which certification of competency, authority, or credibility is presented.

As with state agency inspections, a letter is sent to the lab announcing the date of the upcoming COLA inspection. COLA's Accreditation Manual stipulates their "criteria for quality laboratory performance" and provides each lab with self-assessment questions that cover laboratory operation.

- Specimen collection
- Personnel
- Proficiency testing
- Quality assurance

The self-assessment contains 299 questions for the lab to use as an educational tool to help the lab systematically evaluate the quality of their laboratory and to assist them in determining if there are any areas of the laboratory that are out of compliance with COLA standards for accreditation.

It should be noted that according to CLIA regulations, the state agency is to conduct, on a representative sample basis, inspections of accredited laboratories as a means of validating the performance of an accreditation organization, such as COLA. In other words, a COLA-accredited lab may also have an additional inspection by the state agency after their COLA inspection.

68

CHAPTER 24

Inspection Preparation

State Agency CLIA Inspections

In preparation for state agency CLIA inspections, I created a checklist/worksheet that lists the materials and information requested in the notice of inspection letter. The materials and information are documents that inspectors typically request be made available during the inspection. In addition, I have listed several other items that I think are important and ones that I have found are usually reviewed. Most, if not all, of the items on my inspection checklist/worksheet are tasks I have compiled over the years. On this form I have provided a space to indicate who will initiate a task or retrieve a document for review, when the task was started, when it was completed, and any comments pertinent to the completion of the task. This is an ongoing checklist/worksheet that is reviewed and completed in the month proceeding the "guesstimated" inspection due date (six months prior to the expiration date of the CLIA license) *or* during the last few months of the first year of the new laboratory's operation.

Before the initial or subsequent CLIA inspection, it is very important that the technical consultant prepare for the inspection by becoming familiar with CLIA regulations. The best way to do this, without having to read the actual text of the law, is to access a copy of the CLIA Interpretive Guidelines, found on the CMS website (cms.gov/clia). These guidelines will help the novice technical consultant to get a basic understanding of the CLIA regulations and their application and help prepare for an inspection. Completion of all preparatory tasks may take several weeks to complete, so get started early.

The technical consultant should begin by making sure all manuals are organized and up-to-date. For inspections of established laboratories, this is a good time to toss out any records that are older than two years (shred sensitive documents). Each manual should have the laboratory director's signature and date of the annual review. Each manual should include a list of testing personnel who have read the manual and include their name printed, their signature, and the date of their review, which should be just after they started working in the laboratory.

It is up to the technical consultant to make sure all personnel files are complete and up-to-date. Documentation of education (diplomas or transcripts), training certificates or other training records, up-to-date competency reviews, and job descriptions are all required as part of the employee file for testing personnel.

Prior to every CLIA inspection, the technical consultant must review the following documentation:

- Maintenance logs
- Patient logs
- Temperature logs
- Calibration printouts
- QC log/printouts
- Levy Jennings graphs
- Personnel files
- Proficiency manual
- Proficiency failure corrective actions
- Policy and procedure manuals
- Quality Assessment manual
- Quality Assessment reviews

Despite preliminary review of these documents, things can be missed, or simply could not have been rectified. For example, a scheduled calibration might not have been done at the required time, or QC on a new lot number on a reagent kit was delayed. It happens.

The time spent by the technical consultant to complete these reviews and organize all the manuals and records will dramatically reduce the time it takes the CLIA inspector to review the required materials and information that they want to see.

COLA CLIA Inspections

Generally, the COLA inspection preparation process is about the same as it is with a state agency inspection. I recommend that about a month or so before the anticipated inspection due date that, the technical consultant and lab staff begin to answer the 299 questions as part of the self-assessment that COLA provides.

There are fourteen evaluation groups in the self-assessment questions that help the technical consultant and lab staff to determine if their lab meets COLA standards for accreditation. COLA also provides the lab with self-assessment answer sheets to help the lab staff keep track of what areas they need to correct or improve before the inspection.

The time spent by the technical consultant and lab staff to review these questions and resolve any unacceptable answers in preparation of their upcoming COLA inspection will dramatically reduce the time it takes to complete the inspection.

CHAPTER 25

The CLIA Inspection

State Agency CLIA Inspections

CLIA inspectors are careful not to disrupt the normal daily workflow of the laboratory while they are conducting their inspection. Even an inspection that has been well prepared for can last several hours and require some staff interruptions. That is one of the reasons the technical consultant should always try to be present at the inspection to answer the bulk of the questions and to locate documents and manuals that the inspector requests. This reduces the time the lab staff is called away from daily tasks to answer questions the technical consultant cannot, or to access information found in a patient's medical record. I typically attend every CLIA inspection and reserve a room ahead of time so I can put all binders, manuals, logs, and personnel files, on a table for easy access during the inspection.

During a state agency CLIA inspection, in addition to documents and records to review, an inspector will usually want to see a few patient medical records. Frequently they will choose several dates and/or patients at random. They will want to see patient charts indexed by dates as well as test results for every test performed in the lab for several patients. They will match the results found in a patient's medical record to the same results found in the LIS or the instrument database or on the patient log to be sure the test results were transcribed or transmitted correctly. Acceptable QC for each test on these dates will also be reviewed. Some offices are still using hard copy medical records or charts, but most practices have transitioned to electronic medical records that make this search quick and easy.

An inspector may also want to see the "test order" for the tests they've reviewed, which should be documented in the patient's medical record. Any standing orders found that are older than twelve months would be in CLIA violation and the lab would be written up for a deficiency. This is something the technical consultant *cannot* prepare for ahead of time, but an early memo sent to all providers alerting them that all standing orders must be updated every six months would be advisable. This is especially important in oncology practices where providers frequently write long-term standing orders.

The inspector may also ask for a printout of a random patient's lab report. Every lab report on a patient must have the name and address of the practice where testing was performed. If the report contains results from a reference lab or other outside lab that name and address must also be on the form next to the patient's result(s).

Led by the inspector, the lab staff and the laboratory director (if available) will meet for a short exit conference to summarize the inspection. After the inspection process is completed, advise accounts payable that they will receive a bill for the inspection, which should be paid as soon as possible. The lab can expect to receive a copy of the new or renewed CLIA license in about six months . . . the wheels of the federal government turn slowly!

COLA Inspections

Generally speaking, the COLA inspection is about the same as a state agency inspection. COLA inspectors are careful not to disrupt the normal daily workflow of the laboratory while they are conducting their inspection. The inspector reviews the lab staff's answer sheet from the self-assessment questions with the technical consultant and possibly the lab staff. Personnel files, manuals, logs, and other documents are reviewed as each of the 299 questions is addressed. Questions that do not have an acceptable response may result in a citation from COLA.

Cathy L. Manske

Soon after the inspection, COLA will issue a follow-up plan that has specific instructions for actions that must be taken because of the citation(s), if any, identified during the inspection. This plan is referred to as the Plan of Required Improvement (PRI). Specific instructions are included in the PRI for the requested actions or documents to be completed within thirty days, along with actions or documents that must be completed in a timely manner. Additionally, the laboratory director must sign an agreement to correct and maintain any corrections to the citations and to meet the deadlines for required or recommended actions.

CHAPTER 26

Correcting a CLIA Deficiency

State Agency CLIA Inspection Deficiencies

About ten days after the inspection, a follow-up letter will be sent to the laboratory director. If deficiencies were found during the inspection, the letter will state each deficiency on a CMS form 2567, Statement of Deficiencies. When responding to each deficiency, each respective plan of correction (POC) must include acceptable evidence of correction as shown below.

- Document corrective actions taken for patients affected by the deficient practice.
- Document how the laboratory has identified other patients with the potential to be affected by the same deficient practice and what corrective action has been taken.
- Document what measures have been put in place and how the corrective action(s) are being monitored to ensure that the deficient practice does not recur.
- Indicate a completion date in the column next to the plan of correction for the deficiency.

In order to meet CLIA requirements, the CMS-2567 form must be returned to the state agency within ten calendar days of receipt of the letter stating the deficiency(s). Corrective actions are indicated on the right side of the form in the column labeled "Provider Plan of Correction," keying the responses to the deficiencies listed on the left side of the form. The completed form must be dated and signed by the laboratory director. If there is reasonable concern that a POC cannot be completed and returned within the time frame given, contact the inspector with an explanation and a request that the due date be extended.

For serious deficiencies, the laboratory must submit a plan of correction that is acceptable to the state agency in content and within a specific time frame. Regulations require all deficiencies to be corrected within twelve months after the last day of survey. Additionally, the technical consultant may need to submit a "credible allegation" of compliance and acceptable evidence of correction for the condition-level deficiencies cited. Also, documented evidence must be submitted that verifies that the corrections were made, such as a copy of a diploma, a newly created policy, or a corrective action document.

COLA Inspection Citations

After a COLA inspection, a follow-up letter will be sent to the laboratory director and will include any citations against the laboratory. COLA will help the lab to respond to their citations and comply with their accreditation requirements by providing a Plan of Required Improvement (PRI), which includes the Grouped Citations and Actions Required Report.

- Question number of the citation—from the Self-assessment questionnaire
- Category of the citation—analytic, pre-analytic, post-analytic, or general
- Policy/criterion (restatement of the question)
- What the non-compliance applies to
- Action required
- What documentation needs to be sent to COLA

The customized plan has specific instructions regarding the prioritized actions that must be taken to correct the citations. Also included in their PRI is a Management Summary Report to help in the detection and correction of systemic issues within the laboratory.

After reviewing the Plan of Required Improvement, the lab will need to develop an action plan for implementing all improvements in a timely manner. When this is completed, the laboratory director must sign and date the Agreement to the Plan of Required Improvement and send it back to COLA by the due date stated in the letter. If there is reasonable concern that the PRI cannot be completed and returned within the time frame given in the Agreement to the Plan of Required Improvement, contact the inspector to explain the reason and request that the due date be extended.

Sometimes, during a COLA inspection, serious issues are identified. When this occurs, COLA will request additional documentation be sent within the subsequent six months to verify that the serious deficiencies were permanently corrected. Monitoring these serious deficiencies requires the assistance of COLA's Staff Technical Accreditation Team. If this is the case, the medical practice will be assessed a compliance assistance surcharge in addition to the regular accreditation fees. Obviously, it behooves the technical consultant and lab staff to carefully review the 299 questions in COLA's self-assessment and correct any problem areas in order to avoid unnecessary and serious citations that could result in an extra surcharge.

CHAPTER 27

Top Ten
CLIA Deficiencies

According to the CMS website, these are the top ten deficiencies cited:

- No quality assessment plan
- Annual competencies not documented
- Incomplete personnel records
- Incomplete maintenance records
- No corrective action for failed proficiency testing
- Proficiency Attestation Statement missing or unsigned
- Temperature Log has temperatures not within acceptable range
- Calibration not performed, or not performed at the required time
- Annual calibration of pipettes not performed
- Use of expired reagents or kits

Quality Assessment Plan

Simply stated a quality assessment plan is an ongoing review process of the four major areas of the laboratory.

- Pre-analytical—everything that happens prior to testing
- Analytical—the actual testing process
- Post-analytical—everything that happens after testing is complete

- General review—everything not included in the first three areas such as, but not limited to, continuing education records, job descriptions, panic values, and a record of all quality assessment review documents.

The QA plan should include everything the laboratory reviews on a regular basis beginning with the practitioner's order of a test, the specimen collection, the test process, and reporting test results. This plan should be read and signed by *all* testing personnel when they are hired and/or when any changes, revisions, or updating occurs to the plan's content. The laboratory director must sign and date it annually or whenever changes, revisions, or updating occurs.

Annual Competencies

After an employee has been hired and trained to perform testing, a six-month competency report is written followed by an annual competency report. The laboratory director or technical consultant is responsible for writing these reports, which should include employee name, date of review, and who did the review (technical consultant or director).

Personnel
- Have new employees completed a personnel file?
- Have testing personnel been checked for competency prior to reporting results?

Quality Control
- Have controls, calibrations, and maintenance been performed?
- Have control documents been reviewed?
- Have corrective actions been reviewed for all QC problems to ensure that the problem doesn't recur?

Procedure Manual
- Have new procedures been reviewed and signed?

Patient Testing
- Has direct observation of specimen handling and test performance been done?
- Has the recording and reporting of results been monitored?
- Have the intermediate logs and worksheets where applicable been reviewed?
- Have erroneous reports been corrected and investigated?
- Have tests been properly ordered, recorded, and reported?

Proficiency Testing
- Have proficiency-testing results been reviewed?
- Have failed proficiency results been evaluated?

Instrument Maintenance
- Has routine instrument maintenance been followed?
- Have preventative maintenance records been reviewed?

Communications
- Have suggestions/complaints been investigated and resolved through problem solving skills?
- Have the technical consultant and director communicated changes to laboratory policies and procedures to staff?

Incomplete Personnel Records

Are the following records available for each employee?

- Copy of a valid nursing license, (nursing testing personnel only)
- Job descriptions for director, clinical consultant, technical supervisor (when applicable), or testing personnel
- Training documentation for all testing that an employee performs
- Six-month and annual competency evaluations
- Minimum of a US high school diploma, GED, or a transcript. For employees with high school or other education from a foreign country, their diploma or

transcript must be evaluated by an approved agency for foreign transcript evaluations. Below is a list of thirteen acceptable agencies with their telephone numbers.

AACRAO, Office of International Education Services, Washington, DC (202) 296-3359

Center for Applied Research, Evaluation & Education, Inc., Long Beach, CA (562) 430-1105

Education Credential Evaluators, Inc., Milwaukee, WI (414) 289-3400

Education Evaluators International, Inc., Los Alamitos, CA (562) 431-2187

Foreign Academic Credential Services, Inc., Glen Carbon, IL (618) 656-5291

Foundation for International Services, Inc., Bothell, WA (425) 487-2245

Globe Language Services, New York, NY (212) 227-1994 or (212) 619-0440

International Consultants of Delaware, Inc., Newark, DE (302) 737-8715

International Education Evaluators, Inc., Harrisburg, NC (704) 455-6154

International Education Research Foundation, Inc., Culver City, CA (310) 342-7086

Josef Silny & Associates, Inc., Coral Gables, FL (305) 273-1616

World Education Services, Inc., Main office, New York, NY (212) 966-6311

World Education Services, Inc., Midwest office, Chicago, IL (312) 222-0882

Incomplete Maintenance Records

If an instrument manufacturer recommends a maintenance schedule for their instruments, then recording that maintenance is required. A maintenance log can contain the schedule for cleaning the instrument: daily, monthly, semi-annually, annually, or on an "as needed" basis. The most common recording oversight is not documenting the monthly and semi-annual maintenance on the maintenance log.

No Corrective Action for Failed Proficiency Testing

Corrective action forms for failed proficiency test results are often provided by the proficiency-testing agency. If they are not provided, creating a form is easy. Include the name of the failed analyte(s), name of the testing person, the proficiency-testing event, a statement of the failure or problem, why it occurred, and the corrective action taken to prevent it from failing in the future. It may be a good idea to rerun the failed specimen(s) once you've identified why it failed in the first place. Include the repeated result and documentation to demonstrate that the problem was resolved. The technical consultant or the laboratory director must sign the corrective action form.

Proficiency Attestation Statement Missing or Unsigned

The laboratory director, or designee (technical consultant), and all persons involved in the testing of proficiency samples *must sign* and date the attestation statement. There are no exceptions! It's also important to rotate the person who performs the testing on the proficiency samples. CLIA regulations state that anyone who tests patient samples must also participate in testing the proficiency samples. Even if there is one primary testing person and another occasional person who does testing, that person must run proficiency samples on a rotating basis.

Temperature Log—temperatures recorded that are not within acceptable range

All temperatures that are recorded on a temperature log must either fall within the acceptable range or have a corrective action report written to explain why the temperature was out of range and how the problem was resolved. There may be other factors to explain why the recorded room temperature on the temperature log was out of range. For instance, large medical buildings usually have their heating and air conditioning temperatures automatically set to change at certain times of the day or week. So, in the summer, the air conditioning room temperature may be automatically raised each evening and on weekends, and then automatically lowered each morning. If the room temperature is read soon after the lab staff arrive at work, the room temperature might still be too warm and be out of the acceptable room temperature range until it has time to cool down. Conversely, in the winter, the room temperature may be too cool when lab staff arrives, so room temperature readings should be taken when the room temperature has warmed up. The moral of this story is that you should not take room temperature readings too early each day. Manufacturers of instruments and test methodologies typically recommend a room temperature range that is suitable for specimen testing, so take the reading when testing has begun.

Likewise, be sure freezer or refrigerator temperatures are not taken right after the refrigerator or freezer door has been open for a while. If an out-of-range temperature is read, it might be a good idea to close the door, wait fifteen or twenty minutes, and read it again. It is also possible that the temperature adjustment dial should be adjusted for different times of the year, as ambient temperatures tend to vary. If the temperature dial is adjusted, wait fifteen or so minutes before taking another reading. However, if rereading the temperature doesn't produce an acceptable temperature, it probably suggests that the refrigerator or freezer needs repair or replacement. Document the problem on a corrective action form and include it in the QA review.

Calibration

Almost all instruments need to have regular calibrations performed. Some chemistry analyzers may need some tests calibrated every eight hours, every day, every week, or only every six months. While chemistry and immunology instruments vary in manufacturer's recommendations, hematology instruments generally need calibrating every six months or whenever recommended by the manufacturer.

It is imperative that testing personnel follow manufacturer's recommendations for regular instrument calibrations. Delayed calibrations can often lead to QC problems, proficiency testing failures, an inspection citation, and—most importantly—inaccurate patient results. Fortunately, several analyzers will not allow the operator to run QC or patients if the calibration is overdue.

In addition to performing regularly scheduled calibrations, at least twice annually, calibration verification must be performed on all analytes that do not have at least three calibrators used in the calibration process. For those analytes that have less than three calibrators, testing is performed on known assayed material with low, normal, and high values. The test results of these materials are plotted on a graph against the mean or known value(s) for each level. The calibration verification passes if three or more points fall in a straight line. Hematology analyzers typically do not have three calibrators but are not required to have calibration verifications performed.

Annual Calibration of Pipettes

Test procedures that require pipette samples or reagents must have every pipette recalibrated annually. Each pipette must be sent out to a laboratory that specializes in performing pipette calibrations. Some calibration labs may take a week or two to get the pipette(s) back to the lab while others can get them back in as little as forty-eight hours. So, it would be wise to have a back-up pipette to use while the recalibration is being done. Just as with the actual test calibration, forgetting to have pipettes calibrated can lead to problems with QC, proficiency testing failures, an inspection citation, and most importantly, inaccurate patient results.

Expired Reagents or Kits

Almost nothing will get the lab into trouble more than using expired reagents or kits. Sometimes, it's tempting to run a test on a kit that expired yesterday—Don't do it! I usually ask testers who are tempted to do this to pretend the patient is their mother and ask if they would still run it on an expired kit. Expiration dates on reagents and kits must be monitored constantly so that there is always a new kit or reagent available when another one expires. There is no excuse for running a test on outdated material—period!

As with calibrations, the advancement of technology has made it so that many instruments will not allow the operator to run QC or patients if the reagents on the instrument have expired.

CHAPTER 28

Handling Complaints

The practitioners in a medical practice are the most common source of complaints, especially when a new lab has just been established. They are quick to point the finger of blame at the lab staff or claim that an analyzer's results are wrong. They are convinced that the results are a "lab error" or an "instrument error." Remember that they are often accustomed to the sophisticated laboratory equipment in a hospital or reference laboratory where educated and experienced laboratory people perform the testing.

Until the new in-house lab proves its capability for accurate and timely test results, doctors and practitioners may be leery of small countertop analyzers and inexperienced staff. The best way for the technical consultant to positively impact their perception is to always be available and eager to resolve problems. The technical consultant must be available by phone, text, e-mail, or face-to-face with the complainant whenever questions arise. They must interact with doctors and practitioners whenever possible to demonstrate their dedication to the lab service, to the practice, and to show their commitment to resolving a problem.

Whatever the complaint may be, if it involves the in-house test result vs. a reference lab test result, it is important to make sure that the test was run on the *same specimen*. If it was not, the results will not be an apples-to-apples comparison and they probably won't compare. More often than not, the complaint is that another specimen was drawn (probably on a different day) and sent to the reference lab to compare to the in-house test result. When the reference lab's results were returned, they wanted to know why the results were different. Unfortunately, the test should have been repeated on the same specimen! Serum is generally saved in the lab for seven days so the same specimen could have been sent to the reference lab for repeat testing.

Watch out for a test method used on the in-house analyzer that could be different from the test method used by the larger analyzers used in reference labs. It is always a good idea to compare the result *units* from both labs. For example, mg/dL compared to mg/L could explain why the in-house lab got a result of 9.0 mg/dL and the reference lab got a result of 90 mg/L . . . a tenfold discrepancy, but still the same result.

Another common complaint is when several patients' results show high potassium levels. Once it has been verified that the analyzer is not at fault, it would be a good idea to question the phlebotomist's procedure for processing the blood specimen for submission to the lab. In one of my labs, there was an ongoing problem with critically high potassium results. After watching several phlebotomists draw blood, I noticed that they were not letting the blood clot in the vacutainer for the recommended thirty minutes (according to the vacutainer manufacturer) before it was spun down in the centrifuge. When I questioned this, a few of the phlebotomists agreed that they thought the blood should be spun right after the blood was drawn. Clearly, they got the message backwards! It's always a good idea to make sure that the phlebotomy specimen was collected and processed correctly; if not, test results could be affected.

Something else to remember is that reference laboratory's reference ranges (patient ranges) are typically wider than in-house ranges. This is because their patient base covers a larger population of patients so their reference ranges, or normal patient ranges, are wider. Hence, the in-house patients' result may fall just outside the in-house reference range while the reference lab's result was within range.

One of the most frustrating complaints occurs when a practitioner notices an increase in abnormal results on a specific test.

It's frustrating because you usually need the answers to the following questions in order to investigate the problem:

- How many patients were abnormal?
- What were the names of affected patients?
- What were the dates the patients were drawn?
- What were the abnormal results?

It is important to explain that you would be happy to investigate the problem, but specific information is needed in order to research and resolve the problem. Other complaints may not be instrument related in nature and can range from turnaround time issues, testing that has been performed on the wrong patient, or analyzer downtime issues, to name just a few. Addressing these individually as soon as possible by the technical consultant is very important. Letting a problem languish will not put the technical consultant in good favor with any practitioner or office administrator.

CHAPTER 29

Problem Solving

Before any problem can be resolved, basic steps should be followed:

- Identify the problem
- Analyze the problem
- Utilize data collection and fact finding
- Identify possible solution(s)
- Implement viable solution(s)
- Evaluate solution(s)

How much time you spend in solving the problem and handling the complainant is an individual matter based on your knowledge and experience, your analytical ability, your creativity, and your communication skills. However you handle a problem, be sure to document what you did to resolve it and write up a quality assessment review that includes the following:

- Statement of the problem
- Persons involved
- Data collected
- Action(s) taken
- Resolution
- Follow-up

The technical consultant and/or laboratory director should read and sign all quality assessment documentation.

CHAPTER 30

Medical Practice Change of Status

From time to time, there may be a change of status to the medical practice. Time is of the essence when reporting these changes, which must be submitted within thirty days of the change to either your state agency or to COLA. Report the following changes on the Facility Status Changes CLIA Certification or state agency form or by contacting COLA.

- Change of Ownership
- Change in federal tax ID number
- New facility name
- New facility address
- New laboratory director name
- New phone number
- New fax number

This new information is important for the CLIA inspector as well as for CMS so that the CLIA license renewal bill is sent to the correct address and the correct information can be recorded on the next CLIA certificate.

CHAPTER 31

Moving the Location of an Instrument

Whether the entire practice is moving to a new location or the lab is moving to another area within the practice, the lab staff must verify that the instrument can perform the same way after the move. To do this, I suggest that several patient specimens or frozen proficiency specimens be tested on the instrument before it is moved. Once it is in the new location, QC can be run. If the QC is acceptable, then rerun the patient specimens or proficiency specimens that were run prior to the move and compare the results. If the results are comparable, then patient testing can be run on the instrument in its new location.

If the QC fails, the instrument will need to be recalibrated. When the calibration passes, run QC again. If QC passes this time, then run the patient specimens or saved proficiency specimens and compare the results. If the results are comparable, then patient testing can be run on the instrument in its new location.

Document all QC, calibration and patient results from this study. Write up a correlation report of all test results prior to and after the move, then save all documentation for the *life of the instrument*.

CHAPTER 32

Billing Assistance

The success of any laboratory is not only dependent on how well a lab functions, but also on the billing department's ability to submit insurance claims correctly for the lab tests and to get reimbursed for those tests. To ensure lab profitability, the technical consultant should determine who does the medical practice's billing and if those responsible are experienced in billing for clinical lab testing. If billing personnel have no experience billing for lab testing, then the technical consultant should suggest they enroll in a seminar or other training course that includes clinical laboratory billing protocol.

I once consulted with a new lab that assured me the billing person was knowledgeable about lab billing. Taking them at their word, I didn't inquire any further. Several months later, I was told that, "the lab wasn't making any money." I talked to the billing person and asked her if she was having trouble getting the lab claims paid. She told me she had received many rejected claims that she put in her "denial pile," which was almost two feet tall! Needless to say, she was sent for training on filing private insurance claims and Medicare claims for lab tests. Remember that in the early stages of starting a laboratory, the administrator should fortify an agreement with the insurance companies to allow in-house lab testing.

The technical consultant might be asked for the Current Procedural Technology (CPT) code for a certain test. This is usually a five-digit code that specifically identifies a test and sometimes its methodology. In the billing world, every lab test is identified by its CPT code and not by its test name. Each practice will have a CPT codebook, listing test names with their corresponding CPT code. The technical consultant can be helpful to the billing person by deciphering the correct code to assign to a test. Oftentimes, the billing person will submit a proper claim, but with the wrong code, which would be reason for denial. Billing for lab testing can get further complicated with "billing modifiers" and rules from Medicare that can change every year.

If the billing person is also the accounts payable person, the technical consultant may be called upon to verify that a bill should be paid. The bill may be for proficiency testing, for the CLIA license, for a CLIA inspection, or for the renewal of fees that occur annually or biennially or every two years. Often, because of their infrequency, the biller doesn't remember paying the bill before and will ask the technical consultant for verification that indeed it must be paid. As for the technical consultant, it will be important for you to establish a good working relationship with the billing and accounts payable person, the one that will be writing the check to pay your fee!

CHAPTER 33

Establishing a Consulting Fee

When I first started as an independent technical consultant, I found it difficult to assign a dollar amount to my services. I didn't want to scare clients away with hefty fees, but I wanted to be compensated for my on-site and off-site efforts. Over time, I settled on a structure that has worked out well. My advice to a new technical consultant would be to establish a basic monthly consulting fee that covers your on-site time, your travel expenses, your on-call time, your document preparation time, and anything else that is relevant. Then add to that an additional fee for each major instrument, such as chemistry analyzer, hematology analyzer, immunology analyzer, and allergy analyzer. For smaller instruments, such as a microalbumin analyzer or urine dip strip analyzer, I do not add to my basic fee and I rarely charge any new lab a startup fee. Typically, I bill each lab, via an e-invoice, once per month in the month following my consulting service.

In an introductory letter to the new laboratory director, I include the amount of my monthly fee along with a description and scope of all the tasks my consulting service will provide, including how often I plan my on-site visits. This letter will be sent soon after we have met and they have committed to starting an in-house laboratory. I have never entered into a technical consulting contract with any of my medical practices. I have always believed in a solid work ethic. I have a job to do and so do they; therefore, they should be able to terminate me for not doing my job, and I should be able to terminate them for not doing theirs. My firm belief is that when I attach my name to a medical practice as their technical consultant of record, I will ensure that the lab will be CLIA compliant, and to that end I am committed.

———————

CHAPTER 34

———————

Networking

I have often consulted with billing people from an established lab about a billing problem that a new lab is experiencing. Putting the two billers together to help one another out has worked out well. While it might seem as though every medical practice you consult with is a separate entity unto itself, there is a network of sharing with other practices through the laboratory. Everything from helping one another out when there is a shortage of supplies or reagents to comparing information about a common problem that another lab has experienced. The technical consultant needs to serve as a conduit for laboratories helping other laboratories. In some cases, it can even mean sharing testing personnel. For example, if the testing person in Lab A is going on vacation and Lab B has similar equipment, the testing person from Lab B can perform testing for Lab A either in the evening or on the weekend (except CBCs), and vice versa.

Another way labs help other labs is when new analyzers are brought on board and correlation studies need to be performed. For example, Lab A gets a new CBC analyzer and needs to run correlation studies and obtains blood samples already tested by Lab B. Lab A reruns them on the new analyzer. The results from Lab B (minus any patient identification) are compared to the CBC results from the new analyzer for a correlation study. This works especially well if they both have the same analyzer. The bonus is that the practice doesn't have to send the CBC specimens to a reference lab for testing—and they avoid a reference lab charge. I could relate many day-to-day connections that can pop up between the labs I serve and how satisfying it is for me to help them out simply by getting people from one practice to work things out with another practice.

CPSIA information can be obtained
at www.ICGtesting.com
Printed in the USA
BVHW080030110720
583369BV00002B/210